chance at life

Susan Ellison Busch, MSN, CNP

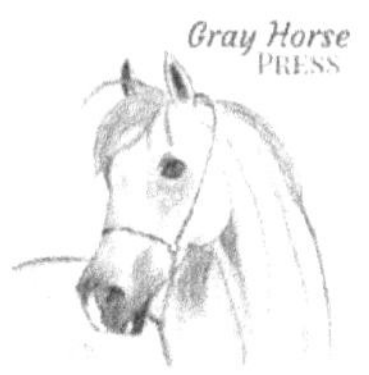
Gray Horse
PRESS

This book is dedicated to people requiring dialysis to live, who have taught me how to find love and laughter amid adversity. They have also taught me to appreciate my own life, the freedom to eat whatever strikes my fancy, and the extraordinary ability to urinate.

Someday in the distant future, stem cell research will enable patients to grow new kidneys to replace their sick and dying ones. In the nearer future, dialysis patients will clean their blood using artificial kidneys the size of cell phones in belts around their waist or with an implanted bioartificial kidney. The phenomenon of a chronic dialysis unit is temporary. In those future days, people will wonder what it was like for the people who spent long hours of their lives in a chronic dialysis unit, suffering inconvenience, drudgery, and pain for a chance at life. This book is an attempt to tell their stories.

- Preface -

Kidneys are magnificent organs that create the precise internal environment to sustain life. They filter blood, removing waste products and toxins, while retaining important proteins and electrolytes. They activate and deactivate drugs and other compounds. Kidneys eliminate excess fluid and/or retain fluid as needed. Kidneys control blood pressure, produce hormones, and maintain a person's electrolytes in a perfect equilibrium. Until the 1970s, over 100,000 people in the U.S. died yearly when their kidneys failed. Rudimentary dialysis machines were used temporarily for patients with sudden kidney failure, when there was hope the patient's kidneys would recover with a few dialysis treatments, but it wasn't possible to dialyze a person whose kidneys had failed permanently on a regular basis without destroying all the arteries and veins in a person's body.

Back in 1960, a kidney doctor in Seattle, Dr. Belding Scribner, couldn't sleep as he ruminated on how to keep his kidney patients alive. He believed that if he could devise a method to pull blood from a person's body, cleanse it, and return it while preserving a person's veins and arteries, then regular dialysis treatments could keep a person with kidney failure alive indefinitely.

He created the Scribner shunt. It consisted of two tiny Teflon tubes; one attached to an artery and the other attached to a vein. A tiny silicon conduit connected the tubes together. Nurses opened the tubes for a dialysis session and closed them when the session ended. Those shunts began the revolution of chronic dialysis treatments. Scribner shunts aren't used anymore because of too many problems with infections and clotting. Currently, fistulas, grafts, and permcaths are used for chronic dialysis. See appendix for pictures and more information.

Vice President candidate Sarah Palin (John McCain) spread fear about 'death panels' becoming a reality with health care reform; however, she was fifty years too late and dead wrong. The United States had already seen death panels. When dialysis was new, expensive, and scarce, many early dialysis centers established 'life and death committees' or what they called 'God Panels'. The composition of the committees varied, but they usually included a surgeon, lawyer, banker, government worker, labor leader, minister, and a housewife. They met to choose from a panel of dying kidney patients, who would receive dialysis and live. They tried to identify the patient who was the healthiest and would offer the best contribu tions to society if he lived. The pronoun "he" is used because in 1960, most women were housewives and though they contributed to their family's well-being, it wasn't believed that they offered much to society. The death panels had strict age limits also. No one under eighteen or older than forty-five was considered.[1]

Sarah Palin's argument about health care reform triggering death panels is the opposite of what happened. Government-sponsored health care under the Medicare umbrella stopped the death panels.

Many early kidney doctors, knowing that chronic dialysis kept people alive who would otherwise die, worked for years advocating for legislation to cover the cost of dialysis. In 1971, Shep Glazer, a forty-three-year-old dialysis patient, advocating for Medicare coverage for dialysis, dialyzed in front of the House Ways and Means Committee. He asked them, "If your kidneys failed tomorrow, wouldn't you want the opportunity to live? Wouldn't you want to see your children grow up?"

It worked.

In 1972, the United States Congress passed legislation authorizing the End Stage Renal Disease (ESRD) Program under Medicare. At the time, there was a National Health Insurance initiative in Congress that didn't pass, but under this alternative legislation, over ninety percent of US

citizens with End Stage Renal Disease (ESRD) were entitled to Medicare coverage for dialysis and their other medical expenses.[2] Today the acronym ESRD has been replaced with ESKD (End Stage Kidney Disease).

Dialysis became available for everyone, not just young, wealthy, white, male, upstanding citizens. For-profit chronic dialysis centers sprang up all over the country. People of all ages, races, and social standings started regular dialysis treatments. Chronic dialysis is also called renal replacement therapy; a misnomer. While chronic dialysis can prolong life indefinitely it doesn't replace a living kidney. Patients on dialysis usually have several health issues that continue or worsen on dialysis.

Incidentally, Dr. Scribner had a patient who was rejected by his own God Panel because she was only seventeen. He couldn't bear the thought of his young patient dying, so he had his engineers quickly design a machine that could be used at home. This girl dialyzed at home for four years before she died. That was the start of home dialysis therapy, which is the preferred dialysis treatment for patients with ESKD, but not the most utilized. Currently only fifteen percent of patients who need dialysis perform it at home.

Though home dialysis is optimal, an outpatient chronic dialysis center is the default. Random humans from every age and social stratum are consigned together for at least four hours a day, three days a week, for as many years as they can stay alive. They see each other, and the staff caring for them, more often than they see close family members. Dialysis patients are at most two weeks away from death should they choose to stop dialysis, or should it become inaccessible due to natural disaster or catastrophe. Most of us ignore or deny our inevitable death. It's not so easy for dialysis patients. They know mortality in their bones. Their lives are spent peering over the abyss.

- Chapter 1 -

Rachel panicked when Michael, the other nurse, called in sick to the United Dialysis Associates chronic dialysis unit. Both the unit manager and medical director were away at a conference, leaving Rachel with sole responsibility for thirty-two lives on her shoulders. Luckily, the day had been uneventful, with trivial problems; one patient complained that his chair massager didn't work, another's TV malfunctioned, and another signed off dialysis early.

The ongoing thermostat skirmishes continued though. Patients shivered with their blood in tubing outside their bodies while the dialysis technicians sweltered in lab coats as they engaged in the physical labor of setting up, cleaning, and tearing down dialysis machines. The techs repeatedly lowered the thermostat settings for their personal comfort, but today, after the third patient complained of freezing, Rachel surreptitiously raised the thermostat to seventy degrees and…so far, the technicians hadn't noticed.

The second shift of sixteen patients dialyzed comfortably on recliners next to their dialysis machines lining the four walls of the unit. Some watched TV, while others slept, read books, chatted with their neighbors, or worked on their laptops. Rachel studied their faces. In the year she had worked in this unit, she had grown to love her patients, their quirks, their families, and the special adjustments each patient needed for a comfortable dialysis session.

Rachel drummed her fingers on the counter at the nurse's station, enjoying a rare quiet moment following the noisy chaos of shift change. It didn't need to be so hurried and stressful, but chronic dialysis is big business, focused on efficiency and the bottom line. Time is money and can't be wasted on leisurely and safe shift changes.

The technicians were taking a break in the corner, talking and laughing about her. Well, she didn't know that for sure, but she knew they didn't like her. It wasn't just her youth; the different roles and responsibilities between the nursing staff and dialysis technicians created a chasm, ripe for conflicts.

It was a lonely position some days, but today the techs had included her in the latest gossip bubbling among the staff. Mr. O'Hara and Mrs. DeLong were having an affair, and two men on the first shift had started leaving the unit arms entwined. Rachel wondered what attracted the couples to each other. Perhaps the attraction was having just one person who knew exactly what they were experiencing. As she prepared her patients' medications, she planned a Shabbat dinner of roasted chicken, potatoes, and asparagus with mushrooms. She hoped her fiancé, Steve, would approve, and planned to stop at the bakery after work to pick up the challah.

The sound of J.R. shouting, "Rachel, Darnell sprung a leak!" jolted her out of her reverie. For a second, she assumed it was just another of J.R.'s jokes, but when she saw Darnell covered in blood with the dialysis tubing spraying his blood like a garden hose, she panicked and ran to his chair shouting, "Oh no! Help! Shit, shit, shit." She stopped the dialysis machine and applied pressure to Darnell's arm to stop the bleeding. He had been asleep, but the commotion over his blood loss awakened him. She pushed the head of Darnell's recliner back to prevent him from passing out. Her heart pounded and her hands trembled with the knowledge that with a few more minutes of this he'd be dead.

Darnell was in his mid-twenties, amiable and engaging, a favorite of both staff and patients. He had sauntered into the unit a few hours earlier, handsome and robust with shoulder-length dreadlocks and smiling eyes, but now he was pale; his skin cold and clammy. Rachel frowned. The technicians helped her re-transfuse the remaining blood from the machine. They gave him saline and oxygen and monitored his blood pressure.

Darnell moaned, "My ears are roaring."

Tamika, his tech, replied, "Your blood pressure is low from losing all that blood. We're working to bring it up."

As Rachel applied pressure to Darnell's arm, she turned to J.R., the lanky middle-aged jokester in the chair to the left of Darnell. "Thanks for the alert." She shook her head. "Close call."

J.R. grinned. "Do you remember the time I called you over for Ali Baba? He wasn't bleeding. He just wasn't breathing. I kept wondering why he didn't move."

Rachel groaned. "His name was Allen Babcock, and don't remind me of that day." She returned her attention to Darnell. "What happened?"

He moaned. "I don't know. I dreamt I caught a walleye off the pier. My needle must have slipped out as I reeled it in."

Mr. Freeman, the patient to the right of Darnell, said, "That was some dream. No one catches walleye off that pier."

Darnell nodded.

Mr. Freeman continued speaking. "That's the worst blood loss I've seen in all my years in a dialysis chair. Are you okay?"

Darnell nodded again, this time tentatively.

The staff worked as a team to mop Darnell's blood off the floor, the chair, and the machine. As it was futile to clean the blood off his shirt, Rachel brought him a hospital gown, but he shook his head.

J.R. quick-explained Darnell's refusal. "A bloody shirt fits his tough guy image better than a hospital gown."

Rachel anxiously tried to figure out how the accident happened. She took Tamika aside. "Who taped Darnell's needles today?"

"I did. Are you insinuating that I don't know how to tape a needle? I've worked in dialysis since before you were born, Missy." Tamika stomped away, declaring loud enough for everyone in the unit to hear, "I'm sick and tired of rookie nurses thinking they know something with their fancy degrees, ordering us around, telling us this and that, looking for someone to blame."

Tamika's outburst eviscerated Rachel. Her face flushed and her already trembling body shook a bit more. Her voice quivered as she turned to Betty, another tech standing nearby. "Um…this machine should have alarmed before Darnell lost all that blood. Um…can you take it to the tech room and check the alarm?" Rachel noted in her head that it was machine number twenty-three. She turned to Darnell. "You need to stay here until your blood pressure recovers. I don't want you passing out at the wheel on your drive home." She asked Betty to give him a cup of chicken broth and saltine crackers.

The afternoon ran its course. Rachel cared for the other patients, administered their medications, and finished her charting while Darnell languished in his chair, unable to stand without his blood pressure dropping. One by one, patients completed their treatments and went home. The techs finished cleaning and calibrating the machines and departed, stranding Rachel and Darnell in the empty unit. Rachel gave him more saline, more chicken broth, and more saltine crackers, but the usual strategies weren't working.

She looked at her watch. "I'm calling an ambulance to take you to the emergency room."

He shook his head. "I'm not going to the ER. They'll make me wait for hours for nothing. Been there. Done that."

"They won't make you wait today. One glance at your bloody shirt and the triage nurse will rush you right in."

He shook his head. "Yeah, they'll rush me in, stick me with needles, and ask questions later."

"They'll give you a transfusion to replace some of the blood you lost today," Rachel offered hopefully.

"They told me in the transplant office to avoid blood transfusions because exposure to other peoples' blood increases my chances of rejecting a kidney, *if* I ever get one…" He looked away.

"You lost a lot of blood."

"I'm not going to the ER. I just want to go home and sleep."

Rachel hated when patients didn't follow her advice, a frequent occurrence in the dialysis unit. She surmised they all had too much experience with the health care system to trust it or anyone in it anymore. "Who can you call for a ride home?"

"No one."

Rachel put her hands on her hips. "Well, if you won't go to the hospital, and you're in no condition to drive a car, and you can't spend the night in this chair, what do you propose…?"

"I didn't drive my car today. I rode my motorcycle," Darnell replied with a feeble grin.

Rachel rubbed her temples. "That's great. A motorcycle." She went to the nurse's station and paged the on-call doctor repeatedly without response. Finally, she reached Elizabeth, the nurse practitioner who rounded at the unit, and explained her dilemma. Elizabeth advised her to send him to the ER and hung up. Rachel stared at the receiver a few seconds, disappointed by Elizabeth's response. She had hoped Eli would suggest a creative solution for her dilemma.

Rachel returned to Darnell's chair and relayed Elizabeth's message that he needed to go to the ER.

He refused again. "Can't you give me a ride home? I only live four miles away."

Rachel had a fleeting dark thought that this was a bad idea, but she was tired and wanted the day to end already. She also needed to get home in time to prepare Shabbat dinner.

She sighed. "All right." She helped Darnell transfer from his dialysis chair to a wheelchair and wheeled him to her car. The parking lot was empty except for one other car and an old red Harley-Davidson Sportster in the corner.

Darnell pointed to his Harley, "That's Rusty. She planned on giving me a ride home today."

Rachel narrowed her eyes. "What a junker."

Darnell put a finger to his lips. "Shh! You might hurt her feelings. Rusty and I go way back."

- Chapter 2 -

Darnell leaned on Rachel's shoulders as she helped him stand and pivot onto the passenger seat. She adjusted the seat so he could almost lie flat, folded the wheelchair, and stuffed it in her trunk. Before getting into her car, Rachel breathed in the cobalt blue sky. Baby leaves in the trees overhead quivered in the cool breeze. Darnell gave her his address in a high-rise apartment overlooking Lake Erie.

As she drove, Rachel made small talk. "Do you have a balcony facing the lake?"

"Everyone in the building does. I watch the sun set from my balcony."

"Nice."

"Nice, until winter when it turns into a high-rise igloo with the snow and wind howling through the cracks in the sliding glass doors. In winter, the lake and sky become an infinite expanse of gray."

As they passed the pier, Darnell pointed. "That's the pier I was fishing from when J.R. rudely awakened me."

"He saved your life today."

"He saves my life every dialysis treatment with his stories and crazy antics."

Rachel smirked. "Yeah, he'll do anything for a laugh. Today when I weighed Mrs. Jenson's heavy clothes to insure we took off the right amount of fluid, he leaned over the scale and spoke to the pile of clothes, 'Mrs. Jenson, I think they took too much fluid off you today.'"

Darnell chuckled as Rachel asked, "What do you do on non-dialysis days?"

"I'm a night security guard at the abortion clinic down the road. Explains why I fell asleep on the machine today."

Rachel raised her eyebrows. "Aren't you afraid to guard an abortion clinic? Too many crazies think they serve God by blowing up clinics and murdering doctors and nurses."

He sighed. "It was the only job I could find. No one wants to hire a dialysis patient. I spend the nights reading and trying to stay awake. Boring. I'd welcome a little excitement like a burglary, bombing, or arson attack."

"Do you carry a gun?"

"Had to buy one to get the job." He looked out the car window. "Dialysis sucks. Death or transplant is my only escape. If I were white, I'd have received a kidney already. White people get transplanted three times faster than Blacks."

Rachel shook her head. "No way!"

"It's true. Racism hides everywhere. Look at the two patients in our unit who received transplants last year. White. I've been on dialysis longer than both."

Rachel wondered about the truth of his statement as she rattled off the standard excuse, "There are fewer African American donors whose kidneys would be a better match for you than Caucasian donors. Have you explored living donation?"

"My sister wants to donate, but no matter how hard she tries, she can't lose the weight the transplant team requires. A few friends from Hiram College volunteered to donate their kidneys initially, but there were too many hoops for them to jump through, and over time, they fell off the radar. I suspect they also had fears about the sketchy medical insurance protections for donors especially with the student health insurance. A few were starting careers."

"What did you study at Hiram?"

"Everything interested me…history…literature…psychology. I wanted to become a teacher like Mr. Ellison at East Tech. He encouraged me to go to college and helped me apply for scholarships. I lost my scholarship when my kidneys failed."

Rachel frowned. "That sucks about the scholarship. The Bureau of Vocational Rehabilitation (BVR) often helps dialysis patients pay for college. Remember Lanetta? BVR helped her get her master's degree before she got her transplant. Now she's an executive in the Cleveland Metropolitan Housing Authority.

Darnell asked, "Do you like working in dialysis?"

"Are you thinking of becoming a dialysis technician? I know a couple of former dialysis patients who became dialysis technicians or nurses. They're the best because they know what it's like from the inside."

Darnell shook his head. "No, if I ever get off dialysis, the last thing I'd want to do is set foot in a dialysis unit. I was wondering if *you* like working in dialysis."

"I don't know…I don't quite fit in."

"Is it because of Tamika's rant today? She's jealous. She talks all the time about becoming a nurse, but she's raising three kids, working full-time, and scrounging for overtime. I bet she figures you went to college right out of high school, with your daddy paying for it."

Rachel shook her head. "My dad died when I was eleven, and after that, it was just my mom and me. We never had money. I'll still be paying off college loans when I'm an old lady."

They arrived at his apartment building. Rachel pulled the wheelchair from her trunk and wheeled it to the passenger door.

Darnell waved it away, "I'm not a cripple." He eased himself out of the car, using the open car door to pull himself up. Once upright he turned and said to Rachel, "Thanks. See you Monday at my favorite place."

She watched him wobble and sway as he attempted the short jaunt into the apartment building. Worried that he'd collapse on the way, she slammed her car door shut, caught up with him, and made him lean on her shoulder. They walked into the apartment lobby with his arm slung over her shoulder. Residents hanging around the lobby gasped when they saw Darnell covered with dried blood and leaning on Rachel.

"Hey, Bro, what happened to you man? What the fuck?"

Darnell replied in a low voice, "Just a dog day in dialysis."

In the elevator, Darnell clung to the handrail and leaned his head against the wall as they rode to the fourth floor. Rachel opened the door to his apartment and helped him lie on a battered brown couch. His apartment was a mess, cluttered with books, clothes, toys, and trash. The sink overflowed with dishes perched precariously. A polished acoustic guitar stood pristine on a stand in the corner, incongruous with the messy apartment.

Darnell noticed Rachel staring at it. "A breakup gift from my old girlfriend at Hiram."

Rachel scrunched her nose at the odor of old food, sweat, and…something else. She wondered if perhaps Darnell had caught a walleye off the pier a few weeks ago and stashed it under the couch. Instinctively, she opened the sliding glass door to the balcony to let some fresh air in. Two frayed lawn chairs watched Lake Erie don herself in sequins as she welcomed the lowering sun. Rachel heard the murmur of voices talking and laughing on the building's back patio as she caught a whiff of barbecue.

Rachel offered to put Darnell's bloody shirt in the tub to soak and get him a clean shirt.

He replied, "I'll just throw it in the dumpster. The garbage men will suspect a murder in the apartment building. Might add some excitement to their job."

"Don't throw it away. It'll come clean if you soak it in cold water. I've gotten blood on my clothes more times than I can count. Let me soak it for you."

Darnell pulled his shirt off and handed it to her.

She noticed his sculpted muscles and a tattoo on his upper left bicep. "What do those Chinese letters mean?"

"Japanese characters meaning, 'This moment, only once.' I studied Japanese for a semester in college and came across that saying. Before dialysis, every moment was filled with possibility. Now I wish for 'this moment only once' every time I set foot in a dialysis unit."

"The moment will come when you like that saying again. You won't always be a dialysis patient."

He told Rachel there were clean shirts in the top drawer of his dresser. Rachel put his shirt in the bathtub, turned on the cold water, and watched the water turn pink and then bloody before turning the faucet off. The top drawer of Darnell's dresser stuck when she tried to open it. She yanked again hard, and this time the entire drawer came out, crashing and spilling the contents on the floor of his bedroom. Rachel cursed.

Darnell hollered from the couch. "I forgot to tell you that drawer sticks. There is a trick to opening it."

"Too late now. Everything's in a pile on the floor."

"Just leave it. I'll get to it tomorrow."

"I'll just stuff everything back."

The pile on the floor contained not only t-shirts and underwear, but a box of expired condoms and a funny-looking blue glass pipe. Curious, she studied it closer until it dawned on her that she was rifling through her patient's personal belongings. *I don't belong here.* She reinstalled the drawer and hurriedly returned its contents. She grabbed a t-shirt, brought it to Darnell and helped him put it on. "I gotta go. Do you have a phone to call for help if you need it?"

He patted his pocket.

She left and, a few seconds later, poked her head back in the door. "Remember to give the Bureau of Vocational Rehab a call when you're feeling stronger."

The bakery where Rachel usually picked up challah for Shabbat had closed. *Shit, it's later than I thought.* Steve is going to be pissed. As she drove home, so many thoughts jostled in her brain. She ruminated over Darnell's blood loss and asked herself repeatedly why the machine didn't alarm. She got an anxious, sick feeling in her stomach when she remembered the pool of his blood on the floor. *I wish he had agreed to go to the ER.* She knew she shouldn't prefer one patient over another but had to admit there was a tender spot in her heart for Darnell. She wondered how he could live in that pigsty and imagined the surprises she'd find if she poked around in her other patients' homes.

Tamika's attack in the dialysis unit still stung. She blamed herself for not knowing how to earn the respect of the technicians and wished they liked her.

She arrived at the starter home in University Heights that she shared with her fiancé. It boasted an impeccably landscaped yard and a *Better Homes and Gardens* interior – an idyllic picture, except for Steve scowling in the doorway.

He expected dinner at sunset on Shabbat. "Where's dinner? The sun set fifteen minutes ago."

"I should have called. A patient lost a lot of blood today. We couldn't get his blood pressure back up and he refused to go to the ER. No one could pick him up, so I had to drive him to his apartment myself. Let's just eat out tonight, I'm tired."

"What?" Steve shouted as he waved his hands wildly. "Did you just say you drove a patient home in your car? You stupid idiot! What if he died in your car? What if you got in an accident?"

Steve was the newest associate at Simon, Zelenic, and Mazzolo law firm and had recently developed a habit of considering the legal aspects of every aspect of their life together, and of course, he was always right. Rachel stared at her feet as the words, *this moment, only once*, popped into her head. She wished those words were true, but lately when she needed a hug, Steve slapped her with criticism.

She missed the funny, easygoing young man she fell in love with. She threw her hands up in surrender, "Okay, so I'm a stupid idiot."

Steve sighed heavily as he pushed past her out the door. "We'll go out tonight since nothing is prepared, but I miss the Shabbat dinners my mom always made. She'd be ashamed to be seen in a restaurant on Shabbat."

"Shabbat shalom," Rachel replied in a monotone as she followed him out of the house. She wanted to point out that his mother never worked and had an entire week to prepare Shabbat dinner but followed Steve meekly. She also wondered why Steve made such a big deal about Shabbat. Friday evenings weren't special in her home when she was growing up.

Later that evening, after they returned from the restaurant, had their requisite Shabbat sex, and Steve was snoring, Rachel slipped out of bed, careful not to awaken him. She googled pictures of glass pipes on the internet, wondering whether Darnell used it for pot, crack, or crystal meth.

- Chapter 3 -

That same evening across town, as soon as Rachel had left, Darnell pulled out his cell phone and called his boss at the security agency. "I can't make it to work tomorrow night. I lost a lot of blood in dialysis today, and I'm too weak to stand up."

His boss growled. "Now, that's the best excuse anyone ever made up."

"It's true. Half my blood was in a puddle on the floor this afternoon."

Darnell's boss wasn't hearing it. "You've missed too many times. If you don't show for your shift tomorrow, you're fired!" His boss hung up.

Darnell's phone slipped out of his hand onto the floor. He didn't have the energy to lean over the side of the couch to pick it up. "Fuck." He moaned as the smoky sweet aroma of barbecuing ribs drifted into his apartment. Any other Friday evening he'd be on the patio gabbing and laughing with his peeps.

He daydreamed that Rachel sat on the couch next to him. He hated everything about dialysis except for the chance she might be on the schedule. He loved watching her work with her curly black hair, green eyes, and gentle competence. His thoughts drifted to his former girlfriend, Tricia. He missed her laughter and conversation. Their relationship failed when his kidneys failed. She didn't consider his skin color a hindrance to love, but dialysis was. He didn't blame her for not wanting to share his dialysis life.

Darnell hadn't given a thought to those humble, bean-shaped organs in his back until they died. They died so imperceptibly that he couldn't pinpoint the moment they started failing. When his urine looked like beer head, he blamed it on all the beer he drank at Hiram. The food in the college cafeteria tasted metallic, but everyone complained about the food. It was more difficult to explain away the fatigue and lethargy that sucked him hollow. Even if he slept all day, he lacked the energy to do anything, even to hang with his friends. He couldn't concentrate on his studies and started flunking his courses. No amount of ibuprofen quelled his excruciating headaches.

There were other odd, inexplicable symptoms too. He had to wear slippers everywhere because his feet were too puffy to fit in his shoes. His pants were too tight even though he wasn't eating much. His professors noticed his decline, attributed it to depression, and referred him to the college psychologist.

He *was* depressed and made the appointment. When he registered at the desk in the Student Health Center, the nurse practitioner noticed his puffy eyes and ashen appearance and suggested that maybe after he saw the psychologist, he should stop and see her. An hour later, she took a brief health history, obtained a sky-high blood pressure, observed the swelling in his feet and legs, and called an ambulance.

In the hospital, a kidney biopsy revealed Focal Segmental Glomerulosclerosis (FSGS). The cause is unknown, but it seems to run in families. The kidney doctors attempted a few last-ditch treatments to salvage his kidneys, but to no avail. He started dialysis two weeks after his visit to the Student Health Center.

For a brief moment the diagnosis reassured him that he wasn't stupid. He could blame his failing grades on failing kidneys. The diagnosis, however, shattered his life. He lost his scholarship, his friends, and hope for a future. Friends from college visited initially, but it was a long drive to Cleveland from Hiram, and they soon forgot about him. He blamed the loss of his friends on his uncontrollable envy. His friends were living the life he desired: partying, dating, traveling, starting careers, and families. He couldn't bear to listen to the tales of their ordinary lives when he was trapped on dialysis three days a week, following a dialysis diet, and swallowing a handful of pills every time he ate. He forgot what 'normal' felt like, and tonight he can't even sit up on his couch without the world going fuzzy. He stared at the crack in the ceiling and asked the god he didn't believe in, "Why do you hate me?"

He dozed off and was awakened an hour later by his three-year-old twin nephews, Clarence and Lester. Clarence propped himself on his elbows on Darnell's chest. Lester stood next to him, poking his ribs with a toy gun.

They repeated, "Uncle Derry, Uncle Derry, pway wiff us."

They wore tee shirts, baggy pants that drooped, and had little two-inch spikes of dreadlocks on their heads.

He moaned and ruffled their dreadlocks. "I wish I could, but I'm sick today."

Clarence climbed off Darnell, discovered Darnell's phone on the floor, and started playing with it.

Darnell's sister Shanita exclaimed in a baritone voice, "Clarence, give that phone back to your uncle right now." She squinted her eyes at her brother. "You must really be sick, leaving your phone on the floor like that."

"How'd you know I was sick? I thought you were taking the boys to the park after work today."

"Mama called and told me to get my ass over here right away. Old Mrs. Winston saw you in the lobby covered in blood, leaning on the shoulder of a beautiful woman, and called Mama. Mama called me and, for sure, all her choir homies. Even if Mama don't live here, she has her spies. What happened today?"

"I fell asleep on the dialysis machine, moved my arm, the needle popped out, and the machine sprayed my blood all over the unit."

"Sounds like some malpractice malfunction in your dialysis unit. Why didn't you go to the ER? Couldn't they give you some blood so you wouldn't look like a sleeping dead honky?"

"In the transplant office, they always remind me to avoid blood transfusions. A transfusion can make me wait longer for a matching kidney, and I'm tired of waiting."

Shanita unwrapped a plate covered with plastic wrap. "I brought you some greens and grits, figuring you wouldn't be cooking tonight. I also stopped at the barbecue pit, and they gave me a slab of ribs for you." She grinned.

Darnell sighed. "You're my favorite sister."

"I'm your only sister, now eat."

Darnell slowly and gingerly pushed himself to a seated position. He nibbled the ribs while leaning against the armrest. Clarence and Lester snuggled next to him, each gnawing a barbecued rib. When Darnell finished eating, he put his head back down on the couch while Clarence and Lester climbed on him again, this time decorating his shirt, face, and hair with their barbecue sauce coated fingers.

Shanita noticed and bellowed, "Clarence and Lester, get over here and let me wash your hands; you're getting barbecue sauce all over Derry." As she washed their little hands, she talked over their heads. "Mama told me she plans to inspect your dialysis unit."

"What exactly is she going to inspect? She visited me once when I started dialysis and had to leave the unit to vomit. Tell her it's a bad idea."

"You know Mama. Once she gets something on her mind, ain't no stopping her."

"Can you ask Will to pick Rusty up tonight? I left her in the parking lot of the dialysis unit."

"Will hasn't been answering his phone lately. We both know he's drowning in the drug abyss when he doesn't pick up his phone."

"I confiscated his pipe last week," Darnell offered.

Shanita groaned. "I'd say that's about as effective as throwing a candy lifesaver to someone drowning."

"Yeah, lame. I hoped the prison stint would cure him."

"Mama has her Gospel choir homies praying night and day for him. She always reminds me, prayer changes things."

"Prayer is about as effective as my taking Will's pipe. Her homies prayed for the healing of my kidneys."

"You know what Mama would say to that. If it isn't good, it isn't the end of the story. The homies still pray for you. I have an idea. I'll drop the twins at my neighbor's, get a ride to the dialysis unit, and ride Rusty back home." She paused and grinned. "I may take her for a little joyride first. I love the twins, but some days I need a little escape."

Darnell reached into his pocket and tossed the keys to her. "I knew teaching you to ride would come in handy one day."

Shanita enlisted Clarence and Lester to help her clean the apartment. "Your Uncle Derry be the worst slob ever." She instructed her sons to start picking up all the scattered clothes and socks on the floor and put them in the hamper. "Try to find what's stinking up this place."

The two little boys padded around picking up dirty laundry, toys, and books, singing as they tromped around. "Derry is a swob. Derry be the worst swob ever." They kept glancing back at Darnell lying on the couch, hoping that their teasing would spur him to chase them around. Their antics weren't working today.

They discovered a putrid pair of tennis shoes, held their noses, squealed, and threw them at each other. Clarence whispered in his brother's ear and they each took a shoe, ran to the balcony, and tossed it over the railing, giggling as the shoes hit the ground.

Shanita heard them giggling and hollered, "Get away from that balcony. You know you're not allowed out there. Come and take a nap with Derry." She turned her attention to the overflowing sink. "It looks like you haven't washed a dish since Christmas. I know Mama taught you to clean up after yourself. We grew up in the same crib. How'd you become such a slob?"

Darnell mumbled, "Why does it matter?"

Darnell fell asleep with his nephews sleeping on his chest as his sister continued ranting and raving, splashing in the sink, and clanging the dishes and pans.

- Chapter 4 -

Elizabeth hid under her covers for half an hour after the alarm went off. "Get up, get up, get up, you old lump of lard," she prodded until finally dragging herself out of bed. Thirty-five years of living with diabetes had taken its toll. Her eyesight was fading, her feet were numb, her kidneys were failing, and her muscles and joints ached.

She thought of her husband, David as she did every morning. He had been her best friend and confidant until he died suddenly of a heart attack, leaving her alone to raise their teenage daughters. At the time, she didn't know which emotion was worse: grief at his death, anger at him for dying, or the guilt she experienced for not taking him to the emergency room when he complained of left shoulder and arm pain. She had attributed his shoulder pain to his tennis game earlier that evening. It never occurred to her that it could be his heart. He was so strong and healthy. She always expected her diabetes to kill her first.

She gazed at David's picture on her dresser, his arms hugging both their daughters at the beach. They were laughing, sun-bronzed, and healthy. Ebony was a puppy at their feet. The familiar picture filled her with nostalgia. She spoke to her dead husband, "I don't know how to stop missing you. Are you still you somewhere? Do you ever think of me? Are you watching over our daughters?" She gazed at the picture of the little bodies of her now-grown daughters and marveled at how the days of their childhood passed like a breath on a cold winter's day.

She glanced at the two blue stuffed chairs in her bedroom,

remembering the evenings she and David sat on them before bedtime. They would discuss their daughters, tell the stories of their days, and share a glass of wine or something stronger, depending upon how bad the stories were. No matter what was happening in their lives, David always made her laugh. These days, Ebony, her old Labrador retriever, took her husband's place in the opposite blue chair as she continued the tradition of a nightly glass of wine.

Ebony was a good listener, but not a good storyteller, nor could she tell a good joke. Cataracts clouded her eyes and her once shiny black fur had become coarse and dull. Lately she struggled to climb onto the blue chair with her bad hips.

Often in her nightly reminiscences, Elizabeth would remark to Ebony, "We're just two old ladies subsisting on memories."

Elizabeth dragged her chunky middle-aged body into the kitchen, and as she made coffee, she saw a Baltimore oriole sitting in the cherry tree outside her kitchen window. His orange and black body contrasted with the gray sky and the white blossoms. She greeted him through the window, scaring him away. She started a new diet again with yogurt and fruit for breakfast. She had a habit of trying and failing every diet known to man. She understood why Eve ate the apple; it was forbidden…like all the foods on all the diets she failed. She filled Ebony's bowl on the floor next to the kitchen table and they munched breakfast together in companionable silence.

Elizabeth showered, dressed, and took a tail-wagging Ebony for her morning constitutional. They walked for about half a mile as Elizabeth discussed with Ebony her patients, her adult daughters, and her fears about her failing kidneys. She settled Ebony for the day, gathered her stethoscope, iPhone, prescription pad, and her reading glasses, and headed out the door to start her daily rounds as a nurse practitioner in the dialysis units. She loved her work, and a successful day for her was being able to make life a little bit easier for even one patient.

As she drove to the first unit, she mulled over her recent lab results. *What an ironic twist. For most of my life, I have cared for dialysis patients, and now it looks like I'm on the way to becoming one.* She wondered how she could follow a renal diet when she couldn't even follow a diabetic diet, and she wondered if she would be able to continue working. The big question in her heart was: *Can I even cope with dialysis?*

When she arrived, she stopped in the staff lounge for her second cup of coffee. A large platter of homemade cookies baked by Mr. Freeman's wife tempted her. The platter held an assortment of cookies: peanut butter, chocolate chip, and coconut macaroons. Elizabeth smiled. "I'll just try one cookie so I can tell Mrs. Freeman how good they are when I see her." By the time she finished her coffee, she had sampled all three cookie varieties. Before heading into the unit, she gave herself an extra bolus of insulin with her insulin pump to counteract the sugar load from the cookie indiscretions.

The moment she stepped into the unit, she was barraged by a multitude of requests from Rachel, the techs, and the unit secretary.

"Eli, you have three messages on your desk."

"Eli, I still need orders on the new patient starting dialysis this afternoon."

"Eli, I gave Larry half the usual dose of heparin today because he bled too much after dialysis the last time, but I need you to write the order for it."

"Eli, can you see Mary today? She fell in her bathroom last night."

Elizabeth paused and asked, "Did you hold her heparin?"

"Of course. We're on top of things here."

Elizabeth thought of herself as "Elizabeth," but everyone called her Eli. She didn't complain. She liked the prophetic connotations of the name Eli.

While the requests were flying, Elizabeth logged onto the rounding laptop. Occasionally it worked, other days not. Today it was sluggish. As she wrote down the requests and started to organize her day, the west wall of dialysis patients, who called themselves 'The Dialysis Board of Directors,' began their comedy routine of moaning and groaning hoping she'd see them first. The ringleader of course was J.R., and they all thought their performance was hilarious. She laughed and waved and started her day at the other end of the unit; she had different priorities. Dr. Max Burnouf would be arriving soon, and they rounded together when possible.

From the outside, Elizabeth appeared the consummate professional, few things ruffled her. No one perceived the deep loneliness, her daily companion, nor could they see the health issues assailing her. As she walked from patient to patient, she managed to forget her own problems and listened to each patient as if they were the only person in the world.

- Chapter 5 -

Rachel had arrived at the bustling dialysis unit earlier that morning at 4:30 am after worrying and fretting about Darnell the entire weekend. The technicians were busy setting up the dialysis machines amidst the cacophony of beeps and alarms, preparing for the first shift of patients arriving at 5:30 am.

Rachel belted out, "Good morning, everybody," as she reviewed the dialysis schedule and logged on to the computer looking for new admissions, hospitalizations, or deaths over the weekend. She breathed a sigh of relief that Darnell's name didn't make any list. She learned that Harriet, the mother of the corner group, was still in ICU. Harriet was a retired schoolteacher who had been on dialysis longer than any other patient in the unit, for over twenty-five years. Lately it had taken a toll on her body, and she was spending more time in the hospital than out.

One of the technicians called in sick this morning, so Rachel added technician duties to her nursing responsibilities for the day. She was grateful that Michael, the other nurse on the schedule, would be arriving at nine. Even with one technician out sick, the day was doable.

She chose to run the corner pod, since it contained only three patients with Harriet still in ICU. Rachel enjoyed the patients in the corner pod; a mixture of races and social networks that, without the bond of dialysis, would never have crossed paths. Jessica was a blind single mother in her thirties with diabetes; Howard owned the Cash Flash Pawn shop and missed dialysis frequently due to "work obligations," but mostly because he hated dialysis. Robert was a retired pastor who peppered his conversations with bible stories and words of encouragement. The patients in the corner group had become family to one another; celebrating each other's birthdays and holidays. They met at bowling alleys or restaurants on Sundays, which are 'no dialysis' days in a chronic dialysis unit. They invited everyone in the unit to these gatherings. Today they fretted over Harriet. They wanted to help but didn't know what they could with her in intensive care. Rachel deftly put one patient on and then rounded on the next few patients who were starting dialysis in other pods, before returning to the corner pod to start the next patient on dialysis. It was her job to assess each patient and review the machine settings before giving the okay to start them on dialysis.

Rachel remembered being intimidated at her introduction to a dialysis machine, with its pump, lights, buttons, dials, spaghetti tubing, and alarms adorning the front and sides. She remembered feeling queasy the first time she watched the machine pump a patient's blood to the artificial kidney on the side. Now, cleaning patients' blood had become as routine and mundane as doing laundry, which is precisely what the first dialysis machines were; jerry-rigged washing machines.

As Rachel continued rounding on the other patients, she watched Elizabeth and Dr. Max Burnouf rounding together. They discussed the patients' labs and dialysis orders. As she watched, she envied their camaraderie. They smiled and joked with each other as they reviewed patient labs and addressed patients' symptoms and complaints. She didn't want to trade her role with theirs though. She had more time to spend with her patients and listen to their stories.

Rachel arrived at Ethel's chair. Ethel's legs were permanently flexed in contractures, she hadn't walked in years and was transported to and from her nursing home on a stretcher. She reminded Rachel of a fragile little bird; alert and aware of everything.

Rachel asked how she was feeling, and she replied, as

always, "Why am I still here? I should have died years ago."

Rachel leaned closer, "You know the answer; dialysis keeps you alive and you can stop it at any time."

Ethel nodded her head. "I know, you tell me that all the time, but I'm Catholic, and I'm afraid I'll go to Hell if I commit suicide."

"It isn't suicide to stop extraordinary medical treatment."

"Extraordinary?" Ethel waved her crepe paper arm around the unit. "Look at all the people who come here day after day, week after week, year after year. Nothing extraordinary here."

Rachel had had this conversation with Ethel numerous times, but today she remembered Ethel didn't have a Do-Not-Resuscitate (DNR) and asked her why.

"My son made sure I had one when I was admitted to the nursing home."

"You're not on our DNR list. You need a separate DNR order for dialysis because sometimes it can look like a patient is dying because of a dialysis-related incident, but we can usually resuscitate them. I'm sure you've seen us call an ambulance for patients in the unit."

Ethel nodded. "Yes, lots of times."

Rachel started rambling, "If you are sent to the ER, everything will be done to keep you alive: CPR, shocks, needles, and large catheters in every orifice. You may be put on a ventilator. Occasionally such interventions save lives, but frequently they doom patients to spend a month or two in the ICU with tubes and machines keeping them alive until they die anyway. I know you're afraid to stop dialysis, but you can easily opt out of that kind of ending."

Ethel grimaced. "Oh God. I don't want anything like that. I pray the rosary every day for a peaceful death."

"With a dialysis DNR order here, we would just keep you comfortable if something happened on dialysis and not shock you or send you to the ER."

"I should have a DNR order in my chart. I'll ask my son about it. He takes care of all my papers."

As Rachel continued rounding, George, the head tech, came behind her and whispered in her ear that Ms. Leggett (who had returned from the conference) wanted to see her in her office. George told her that the cleaning staff had reported to her that Rachel helped a dialysis patient into her car and drove away with him in it. He mentioned that all the patients and staff were discussing it. Rachel's face felt hot, and her armpits got wet. She felt a dull ache in the pit of her stomach and her heart thumped wildly.

The unit manager, Ms. Martha Leggett, was a gray battle-ship of a woman in her sixties, too old to put in a good day's work, but too young for Medicare. She was obese and hobbled around on arthritic knees. She spent her days in her office, munching snacks, talking on the phone, or 'working' on her computer. No one knew what she did behind her closed door when she wasn't disciplining staff or leading staff meetings; she didn't even know the names of the patients in the unit.

When Rachel walked into her office, Ms. Leggett declared, "I am hearing rumors that I hope aren't true, that you drove a patient home on Friday evening, taking one of our wheel-chairs with you."

Rachel flushed. "Um, Darnell's needle came out, and he lost a lot of blood. Um. He couldn't stand without his blood pressure dropping. When the unit closed, he refused to go to the ER…and no one could pick him up. I didn't see any other options."

"I'm appalled you considered driving a dialysis patient home in your car an option. Our liability insurance doesn't cover staff driving patients in their personal cars. You had plenty of options. Just have him sign an AMA (Against Medical Advice) form. What he chose to do after that was his business. I don't think you possess an ounce of clinical judgment in that empty head of yours."

Rachel shook her head and raised her voice, "But he wasn't safe to drive. Even if he signed the AMA form, I'd still be morally responsible, though I guess not legally responsible."

"Did you consider calling a cab, or one of the dialysis transportation services? You could have called our social worker Denise for help. Even the local police department will transport someone in a pinch. You had so many options…"

Rachel felt like an idiot, shook her head, and mumbled, "I didn't consider those possibilities…It won't happen again."

Ms. Leggett wasn't finished with Rachel. "Legal issues aside, driving a patient home in your own car violates all professional boundaries. When you work in dialysis, you need to keep a professional distance. Patients should know nothing about your personal life, let alone ride in your personal car."

Rachel nodded as Ms. Leggett continued, "That's not all; Tamika told me she overheard you telling J.R. that even if he were dying, you wouldn't provide CPR for him. What kind of nurse Ratchet are you?"

"J.R. and I were joking. Ask him."

"Joking with patients is unprofessional. What did they teach you in that nursing school of yours?" Her face was granite as she pushed a piece of paper across her desk. "Here is an incident report for your file. This gives us grounds to fire you with your next misstep. Sign it here."

Rachel read the form and signed it with a trembling hand. Before leaving Ms. Leggett's office, she asked, "Did the technicians discover why machine number twenty-three didn't alarm when Darnell's needle came out?"

"The machine passed all the safety tests. It's possible that the needle got lodged against his chair or his arm and the pressure sensor didn't detect the loss of resistance."

Rachel returned to the unit, her body rattling with insecurities and self-doubt. She had a difficult time focusing on her work and lost her appetite for lunch.

Even though Rachel felt demoralized and insecure after her disciplinary meeting with Ms. Leggett, she breathed a sigh of relief when Darnell showed up for dialysis at his scheduled time. He looked pale and walked slowly, but he smiled at her across the unit. When she assessed him at his dialysis chair, she asked how his weekend was.

"I slept it away in a blur. I seem to have lost my tennis shoes. You didn't perchance pocket them on your way out?"

She tilted her head. "Tennis shoes?"

She wanted to know. "Did you get the blood out of your shirt?"

"My sister washed it twice, still looks like a bloody tie-dye."

Rachel sighed, "I guess I've had that problem sometimes too. You could try bleach or hydrogen peroxide."

"Too late for that. Left it for the garbage collectors to make up a story about."

Mr. Freeman, on his left, started laughing. "Don't tell me you even attempted to get all that blood out of that shirt."

Darnell smirked at Rachel. "I did."

He touched Rachel's arm. "Thanks for giving me a lift home Friday."

Rachel lied, "Not a problem."

J.R., upon overhearing their conversation, clasped his hands coquettishly under his chin and batted his eyelashes. In a high, squeaky voice that echoed throughout the unit, he asked Rachel when he would get his turn for a ride with her.

Rachel gave him a pretend dirty look. "The closest you would get to sitting in my car would be under the front fender."

J.R. grinned. "What a vicious nurse."

Rachel grinned back until she saw Tamika listening to the conversation as she inserted needles into a patient a few chairs away. *Oh shit, she'll be reporting me to Ms. Leggett before the day is over.*

Mercifully, the day ended, and Rachel stopped by the pier on her way home. The sun was a faint orb in a cloudy gray sky. Lake Erie was pea green, and she shivered as the wind's icy fingers clawed through her hooded sweatshirt. She sat on a bench, hugged her knees to her chest, and watched the agitated waves knocking and splashing the rocks. She felt irreparably flawed, a poor excuse for a nurse.

Usually when she sat by the lake, its vastness and peace calmed her. Today she noticed the litter, the plastic straws, the bottle caps, and the cigarette butts floating on top of the waves in the corner spaces between the pillars. She wanted to be a pillar…immovable and steady no matter what was thrown at her.

When she arrived home, she didn't mention the incident report to Steve. She didn't want him to know he was right again, and she knew he wouldn't offer a sympathetic ear to the questions and insecurities roiling in her soul. After dinner, they went for a bike ride, but she didn't try to keep up with him.

- Chapter 6 -

When Elizabeth returned to the unit the following week, she scanned the room as she usually did, getting a feel for the day, looking for patients who didn't look quite right, as she waited for her laptop to boot up. That's when she noticed Rachel hunkered and withdrawn in the corner. Elizabeth, like everyone else in the unit, had heard about her being written up. She wasn't so old that she had forgotten what being a young nurse was like, so she decided to take Rachel to lunch. She called Max Burnouf, the medical director, and told him she couldn't meet him for lunch today.

Two nurses were scheduled today, so it was possible for Rachel to leave the unit for lunch. Elizabeth liked having Michael, the other nurse, on the schedule because he helped structure her day, nudging her here and there; reminding her who needed to be seen in the order they were coming off their machines.

Michael told her, "Be sure to see Marguerite today, she's asking for you." He leaned close and added confidentially, "She made Tamika cry when she wouldn't allow her to put her needles in, yelling that her fat butt would get stuck in between the chairs. Then she had a temper tantrum because she had to wait fifteen minutes for Betty to be free to put her needles in."

Elizabeth rolled her eyes. "So typical. I'll see her when I see her." The background cacophony of the beeping and buzzing alarms on the dialysis machines accompanied her as she started her rounds.

She started with Howard because he looked off kilter. "How are you doing?"

He pointed to his dialysis fistula arm. "I've been on dialysis for twelve years and nothing like this ever happened before."

Elizabeth examined his arm. It was three times its normal size and starting to turn black and blue. She felt its temperature and checked for pulses. "I am amazed that Betty was able to get two needles in your fistula today. What happened?"

"During dialysis last Friday, I must have moved my arm and the needle dislodged from my fistula, and the machine continued pumping blood into my arm."

"Didn't it hurt?"

"It hurt a little, but I'm tough. I have grown accustomed to dialysis discomforts over the years.

"Hmmm…I wonder why the machine didn't alarm. It's going to take a few months for your arm to return to normal. Thank God it didn't ruin your fistula. Be sure to keep that arm elevated as much as you can and use it as much as possible."

Howard shook his head. "Easier said than done. Moving this arm is like carrying a heavy bucket. I don't know what I'd do if I didn't have Tamika's son Kelvin helping me at the pawn shop when people bring in heavy objects like lawnmowers or snow blowers."

Tamika overheard Howard and beamed with pride. "Kelvin entertains us at dinner with pawn shop stories. Last night he had us all in hysterics about a woman pawning a haunted TV."

Howard responded, "Kelvin has a good bullshit meter. Yesterday he called the cops on a man who tried to pawn a stolen saxophone. The thief didn't know that it's possible to register musical instruments."

Elizabeth, perceiving that Tamika had recovered from Marguerite's earlier abuse, added, "I hear Kelvin received a scholarship to Ohio State. He probably got his smarts from his mom."

Tamika grinned.

Howard sighed, "I finally found decent help and he's

deserting me in a few months."

Elizabeth said, "Hopefully he'll be around long enough for your arm to heal. With Kelvin on board, you can stay for your entire dialysis treatment."

Howard glanced away and pretended not to hear.

Elizabeth walked to the next patient, and the next, and the next. Rounding used to be easy for her, but now her legs ached, and she needed a nap. Eventually, she arrived at Marguerite's chair. Marguerite was a tiny slip of a woman in her seventies who lived a pampered existence in a tiny wealthy village bordering Lake Erie. Her mansion had the great lake for its backyard.

Elizabeth knew her story well. Marguerite had not adjusted well to dialysis. Though she had gotten on the transplant list the moment she learned her kidneys were failing, three years had passed without a kidney. Not a single family member or friend had volunteered to donate. She complained daily about the dialysis unit with all its noise, smells, and riff raff. She had refused to try peritoneal dialysis (a dialysis treatment she could do herself at home) because she worried that carrying two liters of fluid in her abdomen would blight her slim, girlish figure. She feared growing old and ugly and had wasted tens of thousands of dollars on facelifts that tightened the skin on her bony face, leaving her with perpetually startled eyes. Early in her dialysis career she had tried hiring dialysis technicians to dialyze her at home, but each quit after a few sessions because of her constant berating and criticism. She was the most difficult patient in the dialysis unit, and Elizabeth had overheard many breakroom fantasy discussions of wheeling her dialysis chair to the edge of a tall cliff overlooking Lake Erie and dumping her in.

Marguerite beamed as Elizabeth arrived at her chair. Her red hair was so perfectly coiffed it looked like a wig. "Eli, I want you to be the first to know that my husband found a broker in New York City who arranges international kidney transplants. It's expensive, but worth it for my quality of life. My husband and I are headed to Mexico as soon as I finish dialysis today."

The revelation shocked Elizabeth, and she blurted out, "That's illegal, dangerous, and immoral. In the black-market kidney trade, the donors are usually desperate to feed their families, and they often never see the money."

"What about me? I'm desperate to get off dialysis."

Elizabeth continued her objections. "What do you know about the donor? What if the kidney doesn't match your antibodies? What if the kidney donor has HIV, hepatitis C, or other viruses? There are diseases in Mexico not found in the United States. How can you trust a crackerjack surgeon in Mexico, that you don't know, to put in a kidney? It could be a death sentence for you. Don't do it!"

"Our broker has arranged hundreds of transplants. A piece of cake to attach a kidney to someone."

Elizabeth persisted in arguing with her. "All that money is just going to pad the bank account of the 'businessman' arranging the transplant. Who's going to take care of you after the transplant, and monitor you for rejection and infection? I doubt any nephrologist in Cleveland would be willing to touch you with a black-market kidney inside you."

"With a new kidney, I won't need a nephrologist. I won't have to look at another dialysis machine or set foot in this dialysis unit again."

Elizabeth persisted. "Even with a transplant, you still need medications and monitoring. Isn't your daughter a physician? Surely, she tried to talk you out of it."

"I don't care what she says. I'm getting a living kidney tomorrow. End of story."

Elizabeth walked away from Marguerite, head reeling. As she moved on to the next patient, she overheard Mattie, the patient next to Marguerite, ask her for the contact information of the man arranging the transplant.

Out of the corner of her eye, Elizabeth saw Marguerite jut her chin in the air and reply, "You can't afford it."

Elizabeth's rounding brought her to Rachel. Rachel had her head down as she prepared patients' medications. Elizabeth asked Rachel how she was doing, and she responded without looking up. "I'm sure you've heard. I am a pariah."

"Rachel, since there are two nurses working today, I am treating you to lunch. I have a few stories to tell you."

- Chapter 7 -

A curious and reserved Rachel slid into Elizabeth's car. She had always admired Eli's knowledge and expertise and felt intimidated to be going to lunch with her. A concrete jungle of fast-food restaurants and big box stores like Walmart and Target loomed around the corner from the unit.

The day was hot, and as they waited at a light with trucks rumbling and cars honking, Elizabeth said, "Let's pick up some subs and steal away to the lake."

Rachel nodded her head. "Good idea. This traffic is giving me a headache."

As they drove to the lake, Elizabeth asked Rachel how her wedding plans were coming.

"Well, we've set the date and reserved the synagogue and the reception center. That's about it. I think there's time for everything else." She didn't mention that she was starting to get cold feet and that living with Steve wasn't as much fun as she had anticipated.

When they arrived at the park, they found a weathered picnic table in the shade. Lake Erie peeked at them between the tree branches. Seagulls screeched overhead, and a swallow-tail butterfly lingered at the edge of the table before unfolding its wings and flitting away. A gentle breeze mussed their hair. They unfolded their napkins to use as placemats as a little inchworm inched toward their lunches.

"Rachel, I brought you out to lunch because I heard you were written up."

"I am surprised you wanted to take me to lunch."

"I'm sorry I left you holding the bag when you called about

Darnell. When I hung up that day, I knew Darnell wouldn't go to the ER but didn't allow myself to imagine your predicament or suggest other options." She tilted her head and smiled. "I didn't expect you to drive Darnell home, but I admire the kindness in your heart. In the grand scale of medical errors, driving Darnell home was small potatoes. I was written up a few times when I was a new nurse."

Rachel couldn't believe that her role model had ever made a mistake. Her eyes widened. "You? Written up?"

Elizabeth leaned in close and lowered her voice, "Keep this under wraps. I have a few 'incident reports' gathering dust in my 'permanent file.' I tried to be a good nurse but made some dumb mistakes when I was young."

"Mistakes?"

"One time, as I shaved a humongous semi-comatose man in his chair, he slid forward in slow motion out of the chair and on to the floor. No injury, just lying on the floor and too big for me to lift by myself. I was a tiny nurse in those days. I pressed the call light and waited for a pair of strong arms. Half of his face was still slathered with shaving cream so as I waited, I decided to save time by finishing his shave. The head nurse answered the call light to find me straddling the man with a razor in my hand.

Rachel put her hands to her cheeks. "Oh no! Did anyone take a picture?"

"Thank God we didn't have cell phones in those days. Fewer records hanging around of my past foolishness. Another time, my assignment was to sample urine from the urinary catheters of diabetic patients. That's how we checked patient's blood sugars before finger sticks were invented. I thought I was sampling urine, but in reality, I was removing the sterile water from the balloons holding the catheters in place. Five patient's catheters slipped out before I realized my mistake."

"Oh no!" Rachel laughed. She was feeling better already.

Maybe every nurse makes mistakes sometimes.

Elizabeth giggled. "I had been wondering why all their blood sugar results registered zero. And then…there was the dead body snafu."

"Dead body?"

"After a woman died, another new nurse and I were assigned to prepare the body for the morgue." Elizabeth pointed her finger in the air. "As you know, dentures need to be returned to the mouth quickly before rigor mortis sets in. The other nurse, Mary, asked me to put the dentures in as she ran to get the basin, soap, towels, and sheets. I grabbed the dentures from the bedside table and struggled to put them in. I had such a hard time getting them in place that I thought rigor mortis had already set in. Mary returned with the supplies, looked at the corpse, and asked why it was smiling. I replied, 'She is happy to have her dentures back.' Mary asked, 'Have you ever viewed smiling remains at a funeral home?' I asked her to help me adjust them better, but she refused to stick her hand into the mouth of a dead person. To tell you the truth, we both had the heebie jeebies. This was the first dead body either of us had prepared and we were a little spooked. We both breathed a sigh of relief when the orderlies transported the smiling remains to the morgue.

"A few minutes later, as I sat at the nurse's station writing my notes, I heard a steady click, click, drag getting louder and louder." Elizabeth rapped her knuckle hand on the table and stomped her foot on the ground to mimic the sound as if she were telling a ghost story.

Rachel waited in anticipation as Elizabeth continued, "I glanced up to see the dead patient's roommate hobbling down the hall towards me with her walker. When she arrived, she peaked over the counter at the nurses' station and asked, 'Has anyone seen my dentures? They were on my bedside table an hour ago.'"

Rachel laughed like she hadn't in a long time. When she finished, Elizabeth waxed philosophical. "Incident reports don't make better nurses. After my first incident report, I felt bad for six weeks, the second one for three weeks or so." She shrugged her shoulders, "After that, I learned to let them slide off my back. The secret is forgiving yourself and learning from every mistake. I became a good nurse, but I didn't start out being one…and to this day, I still make mistakes. Mistakes happen with poor staffing, poor training, or bad procedures. Instead of writing you up, Ms. Leggett could have taken the opportunity to establish a procedure for getting an unstable patient home safely. Darnell wasn't the first patient in this predicament."

"Eli, I don't think I'll make that stupid mistake again, but now I'm afraid of getting fired for future mistakes. Ms. Leggett said the incident report in my file would be grounds for firing me with my next mistake."

"That doesn't surprise me. Many years ago, Ms. Leggett and I were young nurses together. An incident report landed in her file. It didn't make her a better nurse, she became rigid; no creativity, following regulations to a T."

Rachel smirked. "I can't imagine Ms. Leggett being young. She is such a dinosaur…"

Elizabeth grinned. "I guess that makes me a dinosaur too… been nursing since the Jurassic age."

"Sorry Eli, that was bad."

Eli waved her hand. "No worries. I shouldn't have been talking about her."

"Eli, I have another question. Ms. Leggett accused me of not having professional boundaries. I don't get it. We see our patients fifteen to twenty hours weekly, year in and year out, spending more time with them than they spend with their families and friends. It's natural for friendships to develop. The techs often join the corner pod patients for Sunday bowling parties. Howard, the pawnbroker, hired Tamika's son to work in his store. Aren't those boundaries being crossed?"

Elizabeth nodded. "I suppose. Boundaries are just an imaginary construct to maintain a professional distance…quite challenging in a chronic dialysis unit."

Rachel nodded her head in agreement and Elizabeth probed, "What do you perceive as the risks of developing relationships with patients?"

Rachel speculated, "I suppose the biggest risk would be panicking when a patient you love has a medical emergency. Also, patients might perceive that you give one patient special treatment over another…J.R. was just teasing, but last week he asked when he'd get his turn for a ride home with me.

Elizabeth nodded. "You get it. Boundaries also protect you from drowning in grief whenever a patient dies. The most important boundary to maintain is to avoid any romantic attachments to your patients."

"A romantic attachment? That's insane. Who would do such a thing?" Rachel looked at her watch, stood, collected the napkin and wrappers from her lunch and announced. "I'm starting over, keeping a professional distance at all times."

Elizabeth stood, gathered the remains of her lunch, and held out her hand as if she were a traffic cop. "Whoa, not so fast. Sometimes boundaries interfere with healing when a patient is frightened or suffering. At the end of the day, we're merely humans carrying each other home."

Rachel pondered their conversation as they walked in silence to the car.

Then Elizabeth asked Rachel, "Did you know Marguerite plans to obtain a black-market kidney in Mexico?"

"What chutzpah!" Rachel exclaimed. "Did you call the police?"

"I don't know what to do…reporting illegal transplants isn't required by law as in the case of child or elder abuse.

Reporting it could get me into legal problems regarding a breach of confidentiality; you know, HIPAA laws. Even in my dinosaur old age, I still wake at night with nagging questions."

As they rode back to the unit, the conversation veered to their mutual patients. Rachel asked Elizabeth if she had seen Mr. Howard's arm. She told her that Mr. Howard had been dialyzing on machine twenty-three, the same machine that didn't alarm when Darnell's needle came out. "I know there is something wrong with that machine, but every time I remove it from the floor to be checked, it passes all the safety checks."

Elizabeth replied, "I haven't worked with a dialysis machine for over twenty years. Dialysis machines these days are high tech computers; the machines I used were just pieces and parts, tubing, gauges, and pumps. We used a little screw clamp to add pressure to the lines to remove fluid from patients. I suggest asking a tech who knows these newer machines and their computer systems."

"That reminds me, the first patient on my list this afternoon is Darnell. I don't know how he can stand up with his blood count so low. He needs a blood transfusion."

"Good luck with that plan. He is so afraid of doing anything that would hinder his chances of receiving a transplant."

Elizabeth nodded. "We'll have to manage his anemia with iron and EPO, but it will take six weeks or longer before he starts feeling better."

When they arrived at the dialysis center, Rachel impulsively gave Elizabeth a big hug and said, "Thanks for lunch and the pep talk." Her hero was becoming her friend.

- Chapter 8 -

Darnell never solved the mystery of his missing tennis shoes, but he didn't need tennis shoes in the early weeks after his dialysis blood loss. He was so anemic that he had to catch his breath after walking from one room to another. He lacked the strength to shoot hoops or ride his motorcycle. He let his beard grow in because he became dizzy and nauseated when standing in front of the bathroom mirror to shave. He had become a feeble old man, trembly and weak. He thought of old Mr. Watson struggling to walk into the dialysis unit using his walker, stopping occasionally to catch his breath. *I'm just like him now.*

Often during those weeks, Darnell wondered if he had been a fool for refusing a transfusion. *I'm never getting a kidney transplant anyway.* Darnell spent his non-dialysis days on his balcony staring at Lake Erie in all her changing moods. He was sick and tired of feeling sick and tired.

Shanita visited daily with her sons. Clarence and Lester always jumped on him, prodding him to play with them. They didn't understand why he wouldn't play with them. That was the most difficult part of his convalescence. He wanted to be able to play with them more than they wanted him to play with them.

As his nephews snuggled next to him on the couch he tried to explain to them that he needed more red blood cells running around in his body to be strong enough to play with them. He told them his body was working as fast as it could to make more red blood cells, but it would take a few more weeks. Clarence and Lester didn't understand a word he said, but they created a new game of running around flexing their muscles and pretending to be Darnell's red blood cells.

After a few weeks of incapacitating fatigue, he gradually started feeling stronger, more like himself. Rachel had been pestering him when he was on the dialysis machine to call the Bureau of Vocational Rehabilitation (BVR) for an appointment. One day he made the phone call, not because he thought it would do any good, but because Rachel was beautiful, and he didn't want to disappoint her.

Rain slid in sheets against his balcony window the morning of the appointment. He didn't want to leave his apartment in the downpour and wondered why he had made the stupid appointment in the first place. He needed to shave, amazed at how scruffy his beard had become in just a few weeks. He took scissors to it first before attacking it with a razor. He nicked himself in three places and used pieces of toilet paper to stop the bleeding. He looked at the clock and realized that he'd wasted too much time looking for a clean shirt and shaving, so he headed to his car.

He lost even more time trying to find the BVR building in the rain. It was a large, square, brown brick building. *Such an ugly building. They should just tear it down.* The receptionist led him to a room to await his assigned counselor, Mrs. Dettinger. He imagined a middle-aged white woman in a navy-blue patterned business suit with a skirt and sensible shoes turning her nose down at him over reading glasses. He fidgeted as he waited, reading government posters and handouts; wondering who picked the god-awful green paint on the walls.

A woman drove into his room on a motorized wheelchair. *Poor lady is lost.* Darnell stood and offered, "Can I help you get somewhere?" She smiled and held out her left hand. Her speech was slurred, her head tilted, and her right arm hung limp at her side.

"I'm looking for my next client, Darnell Johnson."

He took her hand in his. "You found me." *So, this lady is supposed to help me return to college? Fuck. She can't even stand on her own two legs.*

Mrs. Dettinger noticed the three tiny pieces of toilet paper still stuck on his face, smirked, and slurred, "Nice shaving job."

Darnell, embarrassed, pulled the pieces off, put them in his pocket, and sat on a metal chair across from Mrs. Dettinger's wheelchair.

She told him her story. Twenty years previously, she had been in a car accident with a broken back and a severe head injury. After several months in ICU and rehab, she survived, but felt so useless she would have committed suicide if she had the strength and means. BVR taught her how to do things she didn't think were possible and then sent her to school for her bachelor's and master's degrees. Upon graduation, she took a job here, grateful to be of use, and wanting to give back, so to speak. She smiled and drawled, "Now, what's your story."

Darnell leaned forward and spoke louder than usual, expecting her to also be hard of hearing with all her other disabilities. "I had a scholarship to Hiram College. I wanted to be a teacher." He shrugged his shoulders. "But to be honest, I wasn't sure. I loved learning about everything. But then my kidneys failed, I lost my scholarship, ended up on dialysis, and now I can't keep a job because of my dialysis schedule and other health issues." He listed all the jobs he had lost since becoming a dialysis patient.

Mrs. Dettinger listened intently to his story, nodding her tilted head. "So, what's your goal? Do you want to return to school or get a job?"

"I want both, but if I can only pick one, I'd rather finish my education so I can get a better job."

Mrs. Dettinger spun her wheelchair around, headed out the door, and with garbled speech told him she'd be right back. Darnell waited for ten minutes, which seemed like a thousand minutes, before she returned with a stack of papers.

"You need to fill out these papers to obtain the financial support to finish your education. Nothing happens in the government without a pile of papers. It's a bureaucracy, forms need to be filled out to fill out forms; tedious, but eventually the job gets done."

Darnell took the stack of papers and started paging through them. "So…after I fill these out…how long do I have to wait until I hear if I'm approved?"

"Well, since it's early June, and the turnaround time for the application is close to a month, you could possibly return to college this fall." She reached into the pile of documents in Darnell's hand and pulled out a green form. "Your health care provider needs to fill this out. The approval depends on how quickly you get the paperwork back. We have a few people on dialysis attending college."

Mrs. Dettinger continued with labored speech. "I suggest you apply to Cleveland State soon if you want to start this fall. They'll want your transcripts from Hiram. It will take them longer to process your application at Cleveland State than it takes BVR to approve your funding. At the end of each semester, Cleveland State will need to send in your grades and attendance. BVR doesn't want to waste money on someone who isn't serious about studying. You may have to be on their case to get the forms in on time."

"So, all I have to do is fill out these papers?" He shook his head. "It can't be that easy. Surely there are more hoops to jump through."

She smiled her crooked smile and said, "You don't think you've jumped through enough hoops already?"

Darnell trembled and caught his breath. *What is this feeling? Hope?* He quickly wiped the tears escaping from his eyes. He hadn't realized until this moment how much he wanted to continue his education.

He stood and bent over her wheelchair to give her a big hug. "Thank you, thank you, thank you. I'll return the papers as soon as my nurse practitioner fills out the green sheet."

He walked out of that beautiful building with a spring in his step, protecting the pack of papers under his t-shirt as he walked to his car in the rain. When he returned home, he called Cleveland State admissions office for an appointment. When Shanita and the boys arrived that afternoon, they found him feverishly filling out the paperwork at his kitchen table. He abandoned his paperwork to wrestle and play with his nephews.

- Chapter 9 -

A few days later, Eli's suggestion to ask a tech to help her inspect machine twenty-three gave Rachel the brilliant idea to try to kill two birds with one stone. She would figure out the problem with the faulty alarm on machine twenty-three and establish a better relationship with Tamika. After the first shift patients were dialyzing comfortably, Rachel approached Tamika. "I'm wondering if you could spare a few minutes to examine machine twenty-three with me to figure out why the venous pressure alarm isn't working. You know these machines inside and out. Perhaps we can study the machine together and figure out the problem?"

Tamika shook her head. "We can't troubleshoot a machine while it's in use." She pointed to Ethel. "She's using it today."

"Shit. I had requested that machine not be used again until the problem is identified."

Tamika heaved a sigh, "That machine is fine. We can't sideline a machine because you have a superstition about it. The only problem with that machine is the know-nothing nurse."

Rachel felt the air rush out of her. She went to the break room for a drink of water and to catch her breath. She sat at the table, took one deep breath, then several deep breaths, and thought, *I hate working when Tamika is on the schedule. Maybe she's right, and I don't know anything.*

Rachel returned to the unit and resumed rounding. Marguerite was AWOL and had missed four treatments. She suspected Mexico after her conversation with Eli but didn't want to assume anything. She called Marguerite's home, her family members, and all the surrounding hospitals to get an official update. She was perplexed that none of her family members had called to update the unit.

After Rachel finished preparing the patients' medications, she scanned the unit and noticed Ethel slouched at an odd angle in her chair. She went to her chair and asked if she was okay, but Ethel didn't respond. "Oh shit!" Rachel shouted, "I need help here!"

Then she noticed that Ethel's venous needle was out. Ethel's blood had been pouring between the cracks of her dialysis chair, pooling underneath the chair. A normal machine would have alarmed the minute Ethel's needle came out. This infuriated Rachel and she cried out, "This machine is defective!"

Tamika and Betty came to Rachel's assistance and helped with the re-transfusion procedure. They put Ethel's head down and her feet up the best they could with her permanently flexed legs. They gave her saline and oxygen, but to no avail. Her blood pressure was imperceptible, her pulse weak, and her breathing shallow. *She's dying. Shit.* Rachel's heart pounded and she felt weak in her legs. With a tremulous voice she called for the AED to check her heart rhythm to see if Ethel needed to be shocked. Ethel's heart rate was rapid, but no shock was indicated.

Rachel stood, frozen. *I know I should be starting CPR and calling an ambulance. But I can't, I just can't do it. I know she doesn't want to end up in ICU on a ventilator.* Rachel rubbed her clammy hands on her pant legs and rubbed the back of her neck. Her hands trembled. The techs standing around Ethel's chair looked to her to start CPR and call 911. They made questioning faces at each other while Rachel just stood there. Rachel took a deep breath and spoke with as much authority as she could muster, "She is DNR. We do everything we can for her without starting CPR or sending her to the hospital." Rachel asked for the folding privacy screen.

Betty brought it over and opened it up around Ethel's

chair. Rachel grabbed a chair, sat next to Ethel, and placed a hand on her chest.

Tamika exclaimed, "Ethel isn't on our DNR list." To prove it, she went to the nurse's station, picked up the DNR clipboard and waved it wildly as she announced for everyone in the unit to hear that Ethel isn't DNR and needs to be full code.

The techs roared in unison. "Why are you wasting time? Ethel should be on her way to the hospital by now!"

Rachel's stomach churned. She wished she had double checked to be sure that Ethel had a DNR order in her chart. She wished she had checked the number of the machine before she gave the okay to start her on dialysis. She looked at Ethel's heart rhythm on the AED monitor and saw that it had become erratic. *Shit, she's dying.* Instead of getting ready to shock her heart, Rachel removed the AED device against all protocol and grabbed Ethel's cold, knobby hand with her trembling hands. She watched Ethel's breathing become labored, with longer and longer pauses between each breath. Rachel spoke quietly to Ethel. "I'm here."

By now, Betty, in exasperation over Rachel's inappropriate behavior, called 911 and asked the secretary to get the paperwork ready to send with the ambulance. Rachel rubbed Ethel's hand. She tried to recite the 23rd Psalm, scrambling her brain to remember the lines, wishing she had memorized it in Sunday school. "The Lord is your shepherd. Don't be afraid. God is with you in the valley of the shadow of death. He restores your soul. Goodness and mercy shall follow you forever." Rachel put her other hand on Ethel's chest and whispered, "Safe journey."

She may have imagined it, but Rachel felt a slight squeeze from Ethel's hand. As Rachel held Ethel's hand, she kept a finger on her wrist, monitoring her pulse as it grew fainter and slower until it stopped. A moment later, Ethel exhaled loudly without an answering inhale. She was gone. Tears flooded Rachel's eyes.

When the ambulance arrived, Rachel went to the nurse's station to call Ethel's son. The paramedics and techs started CPR, but everyone knew Ethel had died. Rachel let Ethel's son know of his mother's blood loss on dialysis. Her voice trembled as she told him that his mother was on the way to the ER.

He said, "You better not have started CPR on her."

"The emergency squad started CPR when they arrived."

Ethel's son shouted into the phone. "She has been DNR for the past ten years. She's eighty-nine years old, for God's sake! Why would you put my poor mother through that? I hope for your sakes the CPR wasn't successful or there will be hell to pay."

Rachel listened and explained, "In a dialysis unit, even if someone is DNR at home or in the hospital, we always start CPR, unless we have a 'dialysis specific' DNR order. I advised your mom to get one a few weeks ago, but I don't think she had a chance to do it yet."

Ethel's son growled. "When we placed the DNR order in the nursing home, we also had one put into her chart in the dialysis unit."

Rachel paused a few seconds. "I don't think you have to worry about your mom ending up in ICU with tubes and IVs though. Your mom didn't suffer. She was a dear woman."

The son's voice softened and became choked up. "She was the best."

With her office door closed, no one had known that Ms. Leggett was even in the unit. She emerged from her office when she heard the sirens, just in time to observe the paramedics loading Ethel's body into the ambulance as they performed CPR. As Rachel spoke with Ethel's son, she heard Betty and Tamika in the background jabbering to Ms. Leggett about Ethel's blood loss and death, blaming her. Tamika raised her voice repeatedly, insisting that there wasn't a DNR order.

Rachel hung up with Ethel's son and turned to see her red-faced manager. Through gritted teeth, Ms. Leggett ordered Rachel into her office.

Rachel shook. "I can't come right now. All the other patients are coming off and need their medications, or I'll have more than one incident report to write up today."

"I mean NOW!"

Rachel headed to her office as Ms. Leggett slammed the door behind her.

"What's this I hear about you letting that patient die?" She paused a few seconds before resuming her scolding. "As a nurse, you're not allowed to make those decisions. Neglecting to save someone is murder. You can't play God in a dialysis unit."

"She was DNR in the nursing home, and just recently I told her that she needed to have a separate dialysis DNR order here. She told me she wanted to be DNR just last week. If you are worried about possible lawsuits, it would have been much worse if we had done CPR on her and kept her alive for an ICU stay. Her son, a lawyer, threatened a lawsuit when he heard that CPR was started at all." She paused. "And I didn't kill Ethel. Machine twenty-three killed her."

"Machines don't kill people; people kill people."

"There's something wrong with that machine. I keep taking it off the floor and the techs bring it right back, telling me that it passes all the tests. The venous pressure monitor on that machine is defective. It didn't alarm when Darnell's needle came out, it didn't alarm with Harold's access infiltration, and today it killed Ethel."

"You keep crossing lines and not following rules. I'm requesting a formal investigation of this incident. You can return to the floor to finish the shift today, but it may be your last shift as a nurse in this unit."

Rachel returned to the unit, hands trembling and heart pounding. She couldn't determine if her hands were shaking out of fear of losing her job, or shock at herself for letting Ethel die. She wanted to flee somewhere far away forever. Rachel managed to get all the medications passed but stayed an extra hour after the unit closed, writing the incident report and finishing the ancillary paperwork.

As she worked, her conscience accused her. She questioned if she had been 'playing God' and had just murdered Ethel. Her life would have been easier if she had just followed protocol, started CPR, and called an ambulance. How long did formal investigations last? Would she lose her nursing license? As she ruminated and reproached herself, she remembered Ethel's son's remark that a DNR order had been placed years ago. *Perhaps there really is one? Maybe it got misplaced in one of Ethel's archived charts?*

The unit was empty, so she decided to search for it. She found the key to the closet with the archived charts. Ethel had been on dialysis for over ten years and Rachel found ten volumes of old records. Rachel started slowly paging through the first volume. She was surprised to learn that Ethel had lost over sixty pounds since starting dialysis ten years ago. She discovered the DNR order in the middle of the second volume. Rachel wondered who the staff and secretary would have been in Ethel's old unit ten years ago. She was a junior in high school at the time. She took the order out of the chart, made a copy of it for her records, and taped the original on Ms. Leggett's office door.

- Chapter 10 -

Rachel walked out of the dialysis unit, relieved at finding the DNR order. As she headed to her car, she heard her name called. She turned and saw Darnell sitting on the bench at the entrance to the dialysis unit, where patients often sat to wait for rides, to smoke, or to chat with each other.

"What are you still doing here? Don't tell me someone forgot to pick you up. Not that I'd offer to give you a ride home today…"

He shook his head, "I wanted to make sure you were okay."

He looked at her with such tenderness and concern that Rachel broke into tears. All the pain and confusion that she had bottled up all afternoon gushed out. She sat on the bench next to Darnell, shook her head, and said, "I'm not okay," as she became a weeping, blubbery mess.

Darnell slung his arm over her shoulder. She wiped her nose on her sleeve as she tried to stop her tears. Her shoulders shook and shuddered.

When she had reduced her sobs to sniffles, he asked, "Why didn't you start CPR? The patients and staff are all talking."

"What are they saying?"

"You don't want to know."

"Actually, I do."

"They're saying you broke bad; a nurse gone rogue."

Rachel put her head into her hands. "Oy vey!"

"They're wondering why you didn't start CPR when she didn't have a DNR order."

"Turns out she did have a DNR order. I found it in one of her old charts a few minutes ago."

Darnell gently brushed some strands of hair out of Rachel's eyes and whispered, "Ethel was the most feeble, shriveled person I've ever known in my life."

Rachel took a trembling breath in. "Yeah, she was. I'm wondering where she is now…wondering what it's like to be dead. Is Ethel still Ethel somewhere?"

Darnell said gently, "Wherever Ethel is in the great blue yonder, I'm sure she's thanking her lucky stars you were her nurse today."

They both sat quietly for several minutes as Rachel took a few shuddering breaths.

Darnell asked, "Are you going to be fired?"

"I hope not…Ms. Leggett is requesting a formal investigation. I can't do anything right."

"You do a lot of things right."

Rachel, now cognizant of how inappropriate it was to be crying on her patient's shoulder and hoping that Ms. Leggett wasn't lurking around the corner, looked at her watch, stood, and said, "I better go." She mumbled "thanks" without looking back.

Rachel arrived home to find Steve splayed on the couch watching the news. He took one look at her puffy eyes and splotchy face and said, "You look like a demon. Have you been crying?"

"I let a patient die rather than start CPR."

"You what?" He sat up.

"She was eighty-nine years old, and every time she came to dialysis, she asked me why she was still alive. Today her needle came out, and she lost too much blood. I chose not to start CPR and held her hand as she passed." Rachel continued in a monotone. "All the dialysis technicians hate me. They have no respect for me. They're calling me a nurse gone rogue."

"Did…you…ever…think…that maybe they don't respect

you because you let your patients die? Nurses are supposed to save lives."

"It wasn't because of today; they didn't like or respect me before today."

"Maybe you're just not cut out to be a nurse. You don't have to work you know. I make more money in one morning than you make in two weeks."

Feeling belittled, she mumbled, "I know I don't make much money…"

"And now you'll be facing a malpractice lawsuit."

Rachel shook her head. "I don't think so. Her son, a lawyer, threatened to sue when he thought we started CPR on her. I found the DNR order in her archival chart before I left the unit."

"If you're not worried about a lawsuit, why the hell were you crying?"

"You don't care enough to try to understand."

Rachel walked out the front door as the screen door clattered behind her. She needed to think. As she wandered, she pondered Steve's remark that she wasn't cut out to be a nurse. Maybe he was right? Some days were hard and long, her co-workers didn't like her, and she kept doing things that got her into trouble. Some days were relentless with non-stop backbreaking work, other days filled with tedious, repetitive documentation, and other days just gross with smelly draining wounds, feces, sputum, and vomit.

This wasn't the first time in her life she wondered if she was cut out to be a nurse. She had asked herself the same question all through nursing school. The sight of blood and needles made her queasy. She fainted in the OR on the first day of her general surgery rotation. Most troublesome though were her insecurities and neuroses. With each new body system, she developed the symptoms of the diseases they studied. The psychiatric rotation was the worst. Her baseline anxiety exploded out of control. She became paranoid, terrified that one of the psychiatric nurses on the ward would recognize her pathology and lock her in the psychiatric unit at the end of one of her clinical days.

As she wandered, she remembered why she chose nursing. In high school, her best friend, Shelly, had leukemia and was hospitalized frequently for chemotherapy and a subsequent bone marrow transplant. The nurses who helped Shelly slog through her treatment nightmare inspired Rachel and Shelly to enter nursing. The two friends had a noble dream of spending their lives healing people but had no idea what they were getting themselves into.

Rachel roamed the summer suburban streets, remembering all-night cram sessions studying biology, chemistry, diseases, and treatments. She had naively considered her education complete when she graduated, not knowing that it had just begun. Nursing school curricula had taught her the science of nursing, but her patients were teaching her its art, teaching her to how to see, to listen, to understand. Nursing had launched her into the thick of life, messy daily encounters with human suffering and need. She reminded herself of the times she had made a difference in her patients' lives, sometimes with a word or touch, or other times by averting a crisis. No worldly fanfare or monetary rewards for a nursing job well done. As she wandered, she remembered former patients, the stories they told her, and all the things they had taught her about life. Maybe initially she wasn't cut out to be a nurse, but she had become one. She saw people with a nurse's eyes and realized that she loved being a nurse, even with all the difficulties.

She wandered as crickets chirped, and dusk settled into night. She wished Steve respected her career as a nurse. He didn't appreciate the responsibilities she carried every day. She believed the work she did was valuable even though she was under-appreciated, overworked, and underpaid.

She remembered learning about 'Tikkun Olam' during her Bat Mitzvah preparations, the calling on her life as a Jew to repair the world. When she worked as a nurse, she repaired the world one patient at a time. An old rabbi once taught, 'Whoever saves one life saves the world.' *What about today though...when I didn't save a life but let it go?*

She arrived at a playground and sat on a swing. As she swung slowly back and forth in the dark, she apologized to God for letting Ethel go. As she prayed, she remembered her father telling her, as he was dying of cancer, that all our days are numbered by God before the first one comes to be. She hated that saying at the time, but now it comforted her. She hadn't killed Ethel; she had helped her passing be as peaceful as possible given the awful accident. That was nursing too. And then she remembered the investigation and her throat constricted. What if she lost her license? What would she do then? She could always become a librarian. Books, like nursing, propel people into life's messy questions, and they don't bleed or die.

- Chapter 11 -

When Rachel returned to the dialysis unit two days later, Ethel's empty chair accused her: a gaping hole in the dialysis unit of her own creation. When she saw Ms. Leggett, she asked her if she found the DNR order taped to her door. Ms. Leggett nodded and turned away. The techs gave her the cold shoulder with exaggerated politeness. They addressed her as Ms. Rosen, avoided eye contact with her, and only spoke to her when necessary. She felt so alone.

During her lunch break, she slipped into the tech room. Machine twenty-three sat in the corner. She placed a sign on the machine in big red letters stating, *Do not use!* She fantasized about painting it with the words, *death machine* in black with blood dripping down the side.

No. That sign isn't enough. Even with that sign, in a few weeks the techs will forget what happened to Ethel and be tempted to use it again when a replacement machine is needed.

George, the head tech hadn't been around lately. He was responsible for three dialysis units, and the other two units had been keeping him busy. She opened the company directory next to the phone on the desk and looked up the phone number of the regional director of technicians, Mr. Peter Swanson. She nervously called him from the tech room phone so no one could eavesdrop on her conversation. Machine problems and repairs were not in her job description, and she expected criticism for going over both Ms. Leggett's and George's heads.

Mr. Swanson answered the phone. She detailed the problems machine twenty-three had been causing. Her voice cracked and stammered. Mr. Swanson listened with concern, especially when she told him the machine had been passing all the safety checks.

"Hmmm. That's one of our newest machines. I'd like to analyze it myself. I'll send my men out today to pick it up."

Rachel breathed a sigh of relief and hung up.

She stopped at the break room before returning to the dialysis unit and saw Ethel's obituary thumb tacked to the bulletin board. Rachel took it down and studied it. Ethel's picture was of a much younger, rather stunning woman with no resemblance to the crumpled, bony lady she had known in the dialysis unit. Ethel had been her patient for over a year, but she hadn't known that she was the author of five novels and had taught creative writing at Case Western Reserve University. Ethel had been widowed twice and had a daughter who died young. Rachel spoke to the picture, "I thought I knew you, but didn't know anything about you, didn't know the sorrows you carried." She reread the obituary to see if it mentioned the cause of death and was relieved to find no mention of 'death by dialysis'.

When she returned to the unit, two men and three middle-aged women in professional dress were stalking around, looking official. She watched them take Ethel's chart into the conference room with Ms. Leggett. Rachel shuddered, knowing that the inquisition over her suitability as a nurse had begun. As they interviewed staff, Rachel imagined all the negative things they could say about her. She knew that when a person is loved, even the most despicable acts can be excused, but the converse is true if someone is disliked. Normal behaviors are twisted into something sinister with ulterior motives to boot. That's how her mother had treated her; always accusing her no matter what she did or how hard she tried. As Rachel tried to focus on her work, she imagined being stretched on a medieval torture device with spikes stabbing her back.

While she waited for her turn in the conference room, two

delivery men stopped at the front desk and asked for a malfunctioning dialysis machine. The secretary said she wasn't expecting anyone and none of the techs knew anything about it. Rachel showed the delivery men machine number twenty-three.

Good riddance.

Toward the end of the afternoon, the investigators called Rachel into the conference room. In addition to the focus on Ethel's death, they brought up the issue of her driving Darnell home, and her 'un-therapeutic' conversations with patients. Rachel showed them the DNR order from Ethel's chart and explained the other incidents the best she could. The investigators' facial expressions were indecipherable. She sat at the table with sweaty palms and a pounding heart, worried she might pass out. She asked if they were going to interview the patients to get the full picture, and they replied that they always included the patients. Before she left the conference room, Rachel asked when she would hear the results of the investigation.

"Usually, it takes a couple of weeks, and then we send our findings in a letter to the unit." Rachel left work that afternoon insecure with a heavy heart.

- Chapter 12 -

In the ensuing weeks, Rachel managed to forget herself in the day-to-day care of patients as her anxiety receded. Even the techs forgot about Ethel's death and started treating her as part of the team again. One day, as she rounded, she noticed that Darnell had a Cleveland State University catalog on his lap and smiled. "Looks like you're headed back to college."

He nodded. "I took your advice and went to the Bureau of Vocational Rehab. My social worker gave me a packet of papers about my disability, and a form for Eli to fill out, but she told me to start looking at course offerings. I plan to start in August."

Rachel smiled, delighted that he had taken her advice. "What course interests you most at this point?"

"There is a course about the Civil Rights Movement in the sixties with a special focus on the Hough riots in Cleveland. Mama was a teenager living in Hough during the riots. She watched the riots, the fires, and the shootings from her bedroom window. Hough was the poorest area of Cleveland. Mama told me stories of rat infestations and how they stuffed newspapers into the holes in the walls in the winter so they wouldn't freeze to death. The riots started on a sweltering July day when a white bartender in Hough refused to give a black man a cold glass of water."

J.R. overheard the conversation and piped in, "I was a teenager in Hough at the time of the riots too. Can't say I watched them from my bedroom window though. I was throwing rocks, howling like a banshee, and acting like a crazy man."

Rachel raised her eyebrow. "Somehow that doesn't surprise me."

J.R. pretended to pout.

Darnell opined, "Hough is now experiencing a renaissance with new buildings, new housing, and even a winery. People are planting gardens on the empty lots. Perhaps someday it will become a cultural center for Cleveland as Harlem is for New York City. Perhaps there will be a museum to commemorate the riots and the Civil Rights Movement."

J.R. said, "Don't kid yourself. Some things have improved but many of the problems that led to the riots still exist." He started counting on his fingers. "People of color still encounter discrimination in the courts, housing, health care, and education. Look at the Cleveland Public School System. With a majority black student body, it doesn't get the same amount of funding that Cleveland suburban schools do. The quality of education is usually rated D or F. How can a person get a good job without a good education? It's like starting a race fifty feet behind the starting line without shoes from a muddy ditch."

Rachel listened intently to J.R. He usually hid this thoughtful, slightly indignant side of his personality when he was in the dialysis unit.

Darnell argued, "I went to East Tech and got a scholarship to Hiram."

Mr. Freeman, who usually kept his nose in a book or his computer laptop during dialysis unit conversations, looked at Darnell over his reading glasses. "Darnell, you are an exception. We lose too many students before they even graduate. Very few students go on to college after graduation. J.R. knows what he's talking about."

Darnell objected, "But you have a good job with the Windermere Corporation, and you are on the Cleveland School Board. Didn't you also graduate from Cleveland Schools?"

"Like you, I'm an exception. I serve on the school board because I hope to improve it, but it's a relentless uphill battle. When we start making headway in one area, we slip in another area."

"Maybe I can help change things once I get my degree."

Rachel moved on to her next patient, delighted that Darnell was returning to college. She remembered learning about the riots from her own mother, but her mother's story was from an entirely different vantage point. Her grandparents were concentration camp survivors, and after seeing the National Guard tanks thundering along Cleveland streets on the evening news, they forced her mother, who was only twelve years old, to hide in the basement for a few weeks. Rachel remembered being afraid of her grandparents with their heavily accented, broken English and palpable fear. They died before she was old enough to understand how damaged and heroic they were. She thought of them now with compassion and wished she had tried to get to know them when she had the chance; so many questions she would have asked. She wondered if the Holocaust, which damaged her grandparents, had in some way damaged her mother.

Her next patient, Malcolm, was new to the unit, but not new to dialysis. He had been on dialysis for a year until his brother gave him one of his kidneys, which had recently failed. His fistula still worked, making the transition back to dialysis seamless. When Rachel arrived at his chair, she introduced herself and offered condolences.

He shook his head. "Don't be sorry for me. I had ten years dialysis-free. That was a gift, and I know most people don't think of it as I do, but dialysis is also a gift. Otherwise, I'd be dead. I'm expecting my first grandchild next month and I'm glad to still be around."

Rachel was amazed. "I've never heard anyone so positive about being back on dialysis. For most people, it's a time of grief."

"My brother is grieving my loss of his kidney more than I am."

"I've heard that. Kidney donors can be wholly invested in

the health of their donated kidney, often taking it personally if the transplant fails." Rachel reviewed all of Malcolm's dialysis machine parameters as their conversation continued.

"That describes my brother to a 'T.' Every year we celebrated the anniversary of the transplant together. I still wanted to celebrate this past year as his kidney was failing, but he just moped. Hopefully I won't be on dialysis too long. My other siblings and a few close friends have lined up to get the workup to see if they can donate. My sister discovered that she had chronic kidney disease during her workup and is now on different medications. The transplant team discovered early prostate cancer in my cousin. Their desire to give me the gift of life is returning the gift of life to them."

Rachel smiled. "How did you manage to find so many willing kidney donors?"

Malcolm smiled back, shook his head. "I have no idea."

- Chapter 13 -

The following week, Elizabeth slowly climbed the stairs to the fourth story office of her friend and colleague, Dr. Max Burnouf. She battled fatigue and couldn't dash up the stairs as she had six months prior. She told herself that she was climbing so slowly because this was the last place on earth that she wanted to be. She had seen her recent labs and knew that the rising creatinine meant that her kidneys were failing. She was also becoming anemic.

As she sat in the waiting room a large brick of anxiety settled in the bottom of her stomach. She couldn't keep her feet still. To distract herself she perused the educational materials on the rack next to her chair. There were pamphlets about kidney diseases, dialysis accesses, and dialysis options. She picked up the one about dialysis accesses. She had used the same pamphlet multiple times over the years to explain accesses to patients and family members. *Yikes*. She tossed it onto the table next to her chair.

As she waited, she remembered patients she had taken care of over the years, some of their problems, and all that they suffered. She couldn't imagine sitting in a dialysis chair for four hours or more, three times a week, year in and year out. She also didn't want to do peritoneal dialysis. The sugar in the dialysis fluid would make her blood sugars more difficult to control, and she certainly didn't want to gain any more weight.

Finally, the medical assistant called her name, weighed her, took her vital signs, and had her sit on the examining table. A few minutes later her nephrologist friend and partner, Max Burnouf, walked in, a great big teddy bear of a man. He was stout with a ruddy complexion and a shiny bald head. Most striking were his kind and twinkling eyes. She burst into tears the moment she looked into his eyes. At the sight of her tears, he wrapped his arms around her as she sat on the examining table. He held her as she cried. He grabbed a box of Kleenex and tenderly wiped her eyes once her sobs subsided.

Elizabeth spoke first. "I didn't expect to cry. It's just that I know the road ahead. I can't do it."

"You can do it. I've always admired your resilience. Just take one step at a time. Don't be afraid. I know it is harder for you because you know all the things that can go wrong, but not everything that can go wrong will go wrong."

Elizabeth shook her head. "It's not just the thought of dialysis; diabetes is wreaking havoc on my body. I know the trajectory: heart attacks, heart failure, amputations, and blindness. No quality of life in my future."

Max put his hands on her shoulders and looked into her eyes. "Elizabeth, you and I both know that all the quality-of-life studies done on dialysis patients show that the health professional's evaluation of a person's quality of life is much lower than the patient's own subjective appraisal. You'll find that it isn't as bad as you expect."

Elizabeth shook her head. "Often in medicine, we do things because we *can* do them. We keep people alive because we *can*. Death is not the enemy. Sometimes our medical prowess is the enemy. We've discussed this many times, the failures of our successes…perhaps my time is coming. I'm in my sixties, my daughters are doing well and living independently, and after all these years, I still miss my husband, David. Think about it, would you choose dialysis if you were in my shoes?"

Max sat down, letting her disclosure sink in as he fiddled with his pen at the desk. He tried another angle. "Remember all the dialysis patients that flourished, and you know, transplant is still on the table. Did you call the transplant office after your visit with me last month?"

"I called them, and they want me to lose thirty pounds before they'll see me." Elizabeth took her belly in her hands and jiggled it a bit. "I've been trying to diet, but it is so much easier putting the weight on than taking it off."

"Some patients shouldn't start dialysis because they are older and have other medical problems, but not you. You're too young and too healthy for that to be a reasonable choice. I know you've seen a lot, but I bet you have never watched a patient die of uremia, smelled their uremic breath, or seen the itchy uremic frost coating their skin? Have you watched them vomit blood and bleed from their rectum? And then there is the shortness of breath and air hunger when their lungs fill with fluid. I couldn't bear to sit by and watch as you develop seizures and slip into a coma."

"You won't have to watch me become uremic. I know too much. When my kidneys fail completely, I will eat all my favorite high potassium foods…spaghetti with mushrooms, chocolate, avocados, and baked potatoes. I'd die quickly of a heart arrhythmia long before those other symptoms develop. If that doesn't work, hypoglycemia with my insulin pump is a good backup plan." Elizabeth spoke flippantly.

Max turned red, visibly agitated. He put his head into his hands. "Now you're sounding suicidal. If that's your choice, you need to find another nephrologist. I can't support that decision."

Elizabeth stood, ready to leave, but before walking out she placed a hand on his shoulder. "I understand. I'm not sure I could stand by and watch you die either."

Max backtracked. "I'm not firing you as a patient yet, and I don't think it is possible to stop being your friend after all these years of working together. I don't agree with your thought processes today; but we have time. You still have months, perhaps a year, before the dialysis now or death deci-sion. That gives me time to talk some sense into you." Max tilted his head and squinted his eyes at her. "Is it possible that you are depressed? Would you like to see a counselor or psychiatrist to explore your decision?"

Elizabeth sat again. "Of course, the thought of dialysis depresses me. I am in my right mind though, and I don't want to take an antidepressant and whine about my predicament to a stranger."

"What about your daughters? Have you discussed your decision with them?"

She shook her head. "They are both living on their own and busy with their own lives. I see them rarely, mostly just for holidays, and don't want to burden them."

He shook his head, "Mm…mm..mm," making the same thoughtful groaning noise that Elizabeth remembered him making when he listened to patients. "Where does the time go? I remember them as babies, and then as the little tomboy girls running around with my sons every year at the company picnic. I remember Rebecca starring one year in the high school play, and Lauren as the goalie of the high school soccer team."

"Lauren is now working for Microsoft, developing computer programs, and Becky is a journalist for the *Plain Dealer*."

"So, neither of them wanted to work in health care?"

"It's a bummer because I can't imagine doing anything else for a living. The human body fascinates me, but not as much as the stories our patients tell. Every day there's something new to learn."

Max nodded, "Even if your daughters don't work in health care, they need to be part of your decision. Your choices affect them more than you know." He stopped talking for a moment remembering something. "Maybe it's hard to face the idea of dialysis as a widow. I know the loneliness and emptiness of the days since my wife Hannah died. It's hard not having someone to share the good and the bad times with."

Elizabeth looked affectionately at him. "I know you know. Losing Hannah was such a loss. She was so vibrant and alive. How are your sons doing these days?"

"My eldest son Joe is a Navy Seal; my younger son Mark is a schoolteacher. They are as different as night and day."

Elizabeth shook her head. "We must have scared our offspring from going into healthcare."

"Back to the issue at hand, if you were a 'compliant' patient, hanging on to my every pronouncement, I would send you to a vascular surgeon this week to create a dialysis access, but since today you're adamant about not starting dialysis, I can wait for you to change your mind. Today I'll increase your blood pressure medication. Your blood pressure is creeping up."

Elizabeth shook her head. "My blood pressures are fine at home. They are just high today because you're telling me it's time to get an access."

Max smiled. "I suspect you're right. The only change I'm asking you to make today is to discuss your plans with Lauren and Becky before your next visit."

Elizabeth nodded. "I'll see you then, and I'll see you Thursday at the dialysis unit."

Elizabeth walked out of Max's office building into a mid-July thunderstorm. Of course, she left her umbrella in the car. She ran to her car and got drenched. As she drove home, her thoughts swished back and forth with the windshield wipers.

She was surprised at Max's reaction. She had expected him to support her in the decision. He of all people, knew the trajectory. He was right about her being afraid. She wasn't afraid of death, but afraid of blindness, afraid of losing a leg, afraid of having her daughters push her around in a wheelchair. She *was* afraid to discuss her decision with her daughters. They would neither approve nor understand. She imagined Becky's temper tantrum and shook her head.

She pulled into the driveway of a compact brick colonial, her home for the past thirty years. She stopped the car at the end of the driveway to pick up a few fallen tree branches from the thunderstorm. Her clothes were already soaked, but it was a warm summer rain.

She looked at her silent house and wondered why Ebony wasn't barking. She always barked when someone pulled into the driveway. When Ebony didn't greet her at the door, she panicked and ran through the house, calling her name. She found her on the bedroom floor next to her blue chair, cold and lifeless. Elizabeth moaned, screamed, and knelt next to Ebony's cold, hard body, weeping uncontrollably.

She wailed through her sobs, "Ebony. Ebony. My friend. You didn't give me a chance to say goodbye. You weren't allowed to die…You kept me safe with your barking anytime someone came up the walk. OOOHH, I'll never hear your bark again."

Elizabeth wept uncontrollably as she remembered the little details about Ebony. The way she tilted her head just so, how she'd jump in every river, pond, and lake, how she'd steal food left on the counter, how she chased squirrels and followed her daughters around the house when they were little. Elizabeth fell asleep weeping with her head on Ebony's cold, hard stomach, and as she slept, her insulin pump continued pumping insulin into her body. Her blood sugar dropped precipitously, and Elizabeth slipped into unconsciousness.

- Chapter 14 -

The following morning was Elizabeth's day to round, and when she didn't show up by 9:00 am, Rachel started to worry. Eli always called when she was running late.

She called Eli's home phone, then her cell phone; no answer. Her apprehension intensified. Her gut churned. When a patient doesn't show for dialysis and staff can't contact them, the nurses call the police to do a welfare check. She had never done this for a fellow professional…and yet…she remembered Eli telling her in one of their conversations about the importance of a nurse listening to her gut, so she called the police.

The police broke into Elizabeth's home and found her non-responsive but breathing and alive, with her head on her dead dog's stomach. They called the emergency squad who immediately started an IV and administered dextrose. Elizabeth woke and started crying again when she saw Ebony's dead body. The paramedics transported her to the emergency room. The emergency room secretary called Dr. Burnouf when she saw in the electronic medical record that Elizabeth had seen him the previous afternoon. In the emergency room they gave Elizabeth more IV fluid, did an EKG, sent her blood for lab tests, and gave her breakfast.

She felt foolish and ashamed over her hypoglycemic reaction. "I'm a nurse practitioner. How could I have let this happen?" She examined her cell phone and saw the blood glucose sensor had stopped working. She berated herself for forgetting to change it a few days ago.

Elizabeth called her daughters to let them know about Ebony's death, her hypoglycemic reaction, and emergency room status. Both daughters cried when they heard of Ebony's death, which started Elizabeth crying again. Over the phone they planned a burial service for Ebony that evening. Her daughters would come over after work with their boyfriends to help carry Ebony outside and bury her. Lauren volunteered to drive her home from the emergency room.

Elizabeth tried to watch TV as she waited for discharge, but found the silly talk shows boring. They brought her lunch but still no discharge order. No one checked her blood sugars either. The nurse call light went unanswered. She needed to get home, restart her insulin pump, attach a new sensor, and regulate her blood sugars. Lauren would arrive in forty-five minutes to drive her home. Elizabeth started dressing but couldn't get her arm through one shirt sleeve because of the IV still in her arm. She saw a box of sterile gauze on the counter and decided to take her IV out to save a few minutes when she was discharged.

Elizabeth had gotten her shirt and clothes on and was holding the IV site with gauze when she glanced up to see one angry Max Burnouf standing inside the curtain of her ER cubicle. His was redder than the previous day when she told him she wasn't going to do dialysis. He started yelling. "I can't believe you attempted suicide right after your visit with me! I didn't know that you were that serious, that desperate! Why didn't you tell me? That is not the way to do it!"

Elizabeth had never heard him yell before, and up to this point in their friendship, didn't know he was capable of yelling. His angry outburst started her crying all over again.

"It wasn't a suicide attempt," she protested between sobs. "It was an accident. After I got home from seeing you, I found our dog Ebony dead in my bedroom. She was a puppy when David died and was the glue that held our family together in those early years when we missed him so much. I fell asleep crying and forgot to eat dinner. It was an accident. I didn't do it on purpose. I am not suicidal. I may not want to do dialysis, but I do want to live now, this moment, today."

Max just stood there, arms folded across his chest, and shaking his head. He wasn't convinced. "I'm admitting you to the psychiatric ward for observation and evaluation."

Elizabeth shook her head. "Max, that isn't necessary. Trust me. It wasn't a suicide attempt. I need to get home. My daughters and their boyfriends are coming over to bury Ebony." Elizabeth single-handedly put a band-aid over the IV site.

"You need to stay here. Your daughters and their boyfriends can dispose of Ebony without you."

"Dispose?" Elizabeth let out an exasperated sigh. "We are not going to *dispose* of Ebony. You don't understand, Ebony was part of our family. She needs a decent dog burial, and I need to be a part of it."

"You need to stay for a full psychological evaluation."

"I thought we were friends and that you knew me."

"I thought I knew you too, but now I am not so sure..."

The nurse walked in on their argument to see Elizabeth kneeling beside her ER cart gathering her belongings from the shelf below it. She told Elizabeth that Dr. Burnouf was admitting her for observation. Elizabeth replied that the plans had changed. The nurse looked from Dr. Burnouf's red face and crossed arms to Elizabeth who was putting her shoes and socks on. The nurse told Elizabeth that she would need to sign an AMA (Against Medical Advice) form if she insisted on going home. Elizabeth agreed, and an angry Max stomped out of the room.

The nurse returned with the form and, as Elizabeth signed

it, she shook her head and said, "I've worked with Max for years. He's my friend. I don't know what's gotten into him. I'm calling him Mad Max the next time I see him."

- Chapter 15 -

Back at the dialysis unit, Rachel fretted the entire day over Eli as she worked. The police had told her that Eli was taken to the hospital. When Rachel finished her shift, she drove to the hospital and discovered that Eli wasn't there. No one would give her information about Elizabeth, not even if she were alive or dead, due to HIPAA laws. Rachel panicked. She pulled out her phone, looked up Elizabeth's address, and drove to her house in a middle-class neighborhood in Shaker Heights. She found several cars parked in her driveway. *Shit. She's dead. God, I'm going to miss her.* Rachel's eyes filled with tears, and she decided that she didn't belong there. As she turned her car around, Elizabeth ran out the front door and waved for her to come in.

When Rachel climbed out of her car, Elizabeth gave her a big hug. "Thank you. The paramedics told me that a nurse from the dialysis unit called for a welfare check on me. I knew it was you. I was unconscious from a low blood sugar when the paramedics found me."

Rachel started crying. "I worried all day, and then when you weren't in the hospital, I assumed the worst…and then when I saw all the cars in the driveway…well, I thought they were mourners."

Elizabeth started crying again when she saw Rachel cry. Her grief over Ebony was still fresh. Tears bubbled below the surface, ready to flow with the slightest trigger.

"They *are* mourners. Ebony, our dog, died yesterday, and my two daughters and their boyfriends are digging a hole to bury her behind the garage." Elizabeth grabbed her arm and directed her into the kitchen. "After we bury Ebony, we'll eat supper together. I picked up a few trays from Heinen's." She gestured to a lavish display of food on the kitchen table. "As you can see, there is enough food here to feed a convention. Please stay and eat with us. Call your fiancé and see if he can come too. I'd love to meet him."

Rachel pulled her phone from her purse and told Steve the story of Eli's low blood sugar, her ER visit, her dog's death, burial plans, and finally the invitation for supper. Steve told her that he had other plans already and that burying a dog in the backyard was illegal. He made fun of the idea of sitting Shiva for a dog. When he objected that the food probably wasn't Kosher, Rachel raised her voice.

"No, it's probably not Kosher…You only eat Kosher when it's convenient."

Rachel frowned as she clicked off the phone and looked at Elizabeth, "He's busy and can't come."

Elizabeth said, "I overheard the part about not being Kosher. I have paper plates and can pick up some Kosher food for him at the corner deli."

"He was just building his case. He thinks it's stupid to sit Shiva for a dog," she mumbled.

Elizabeth shook her head. "Max didn't understand the grief over losing Ebony earlier today either. Did Steve have a dog growing up?"

"No, neither of us grew up with pets."

Elizabeth nodded, "Maybe he needs a dog. A pet can crack open a tender place in a person's heart."

The back door burst open, and a muddy young woman yelled from the back stoop that everything was ready for the burial service.

Elizabeth grabbed Rachel's hand, saying, "Come with me."

Rachel followed Elizabeth behind the garage to find two mud-spattered women and two muddy men with shovels standing over a hole with a large, stiff black lab at their feet. The women were crying, their tears leaving muddy rivers on their faces.

"The rain yesterday afternoon and this morning made the mud so heavy I can barely lift my shovel!" the tall blonde daughter exclaimed.

"Meet Rachel, the nurse who saved my life today. Rachel, this is Lauren, my oldest daughter and her boyfriend Phil, and this is my daughter Becky and her boyfriend Joe." Elizabeth pointed to Becky, who was short and stocky with untamable curly brown hair.

Both women smiled.

Lauren waved. "We'd hug you, but then you'd be as muddy as we are."

Rachel waved back. "Happy to pass on the mud hug."

Becky handed out papers for a dog funeral to everyone before officiating the service. "Father, your son taught us that although five sparrows can be sold for two pennies, you remember them. We know you loved Ebony. We loved her and will always remember her. We ask you to comfort us in our loss, that we may be able to comfort others in their losses."

Then her daughters elaborated on how much they had trusted Ebony to keep their mom safe when they were away at college and now living on their own.

Together, the four muddy people hoisted Ebony's remains into the muddy hole. Ebony's stiff, hard body fell with a thud. They threw her collar and tags into the grave and added an old bone, her chew toys, and some socks and underwear chewed beyond recognition. Lauren threw in a frisbee and a tennis ball.

Becky threw in an old doll that she had rescued from Ebony's jaws when she was little. She whispered, "I wish I had given you this doll when you could have had some fun with it."

They took turns shoveling the mud into the hole before

putting rocks on top and discussing a marker for Ebony's grave in the future. In the garage they washed their hands and faces in the set tub and exchanged their muddy clothes for a clean change of clothes before entering the kitchen. After filling their plates at the kitchen table, they moved to the dining room to eat. Rachel was quiet and reserved as she listened to the banter of Elizabeth's family.

Once seated, Becky asked, "Do you think there's a dog Heaven? Or do dogs go to people Heaven? I want to believe that Daddy was there to welcome Ebony when she died. I bet she isn't an old dog in heaven…"

No one knew the answers to her questions except to say that they wondered and wished the same things. They all agreed that it would not be heaven without Ebony, so she had to be there.

Lauren thanked Rachel for saving her mother's life. "It's hard enough losing a pet, but I don't know what we'd do if we'd lost Mom too."

Rachel replied, "I don't know what I'd do without your mom either. I suspect I would have given up nursing and taken a job as a librarian somewhere."

"One of us needs to move in with Mom to make sure this doesn't happen again," Becky said.

"No one is moving in with me," Elizabeth insisted. "What happened last night was a fluke. It is not every day that Ebony dies. Have you ever known me to forget to eat? I'll die someday, but you won't be getting rid of me anytime soon."

Lauren asked, "What happened to your continuous glucose monitor sensor?"

"It only lasts two weeks and I forgot to change it the other day."

Lauren leaned her elbows on the table. "That's a problem. We need a back-up system."

Becky's boyfriend Joe waved the chicken drumstick he

had been chewing. "I heard that dogs can be trained to smell a low blood sugar and alert their master."

Becky became animated. "Mom, you could get a diabetic help dog! They just assigned me to be a reporter for Health and Fitness news for the *Plain Dealer*. Perhaps they'll let me research an article about diabetic help dogs."

Lauren asked Becky, "When were you switched from the local news beat? I thought you liked it."

"I loved it, but nobody reads the newspaper anymore, so they're cutting back on all the departments. Now, instead of covering local news, they want me to research and write one long feature about medicine, wellness, or health every week."

"Things are getting leaner and leaner at Microsoft too," Lauren piped in. "They think programmers are CPUs, forgetting our human brains have limits to speed and efficiency."

Her boyfriend Phil, who also worked for Microsoft, nodded his head.

Driving home that night, Rachel felt sad that Steve had chosen not to come. She entered her house to find Steve engrossed in another Cleveland Indians baseball game. He didn't look up. When she sat next to him to talk about her day, he waved her away, stating that the bases were loaded. She went to bed because she had to get up at 3:30 am for first shift the next day. A dark pit of loneliness settled in her stomach.

- Chapter 16 -

In August, Darnell started his semester at Cleveland State. As Rachel rounded on her patients, she noticed J.R. craning his neck towards an open textbook on Darnell's lap.

"I thought you were going to take a class on the Hough riots in the sixties. That would have been a real class," J.R. needled Darnell. "Art history is for sissies."

Darnell responded to his razzing by holding up paintings of naked ladies.

J.R. smiled and nodded. "Ahh, a much more enjoyable course than the Hough Rebellion."

Darnell opened the textbook to a double-page, full-color nude painting of "Venus of Urbino" by Titian. He looked at J.R. and grinned.

J.R.'s eyes opened wide, and he exclaimed, "I didn't know they had *Playboy* centerfolds in art history books!" He then spoke to Darnell in a low, sexy voice, loud enough for Rachel to hear, "Ooh La, la! That looks like Rachel in the nude."

Rachel overheard J.R.'s comment about looking like Venus and glanced over at the full-color picture of the naked beauty on Darnell's lap and blushed.

When Darnell saw her blush, he turned to J.R. "J.R., have you no decency whatsoever?"

Mr. Freeman looked up from his laptop and craned his neck to see the picture. He snickered, "Well at least she has one hand covering her coochie." The three grown men in their dialysis chairs giggled like seventh graders.

By this time Rachel had recovered her bearings. "I am going to separate the three of you for sexual harassment and disturbing the unit."

J.R. replied without a beat, "You old battle-axe."

Darnell snorted. "You're calling Rachel a battle-axe? You haven't met my Mama."

Tamika, working close by, muttered under her breath so a few patients could hear. "Rachel is a battle-axe floozy who kills patients."

Rachel pretended not to hear.

Mr. Freeman chimed in, "Speaking of bad behaviors, where is Marguerite? She was the queen of dialysis unit misbehavior. I miss the drama. Maybe she's on one of those dialysis cruises again. That woman travels more than a *National Geographic* Photographer."

Rachel replied honestly, "I have no idea where she is."

J.R. probed, "If a patient doesn't show for dialysis, don't you call their house and all the hospitals in town to find where they've landed?"

"Of course. We're always checking on you guys. She isn't to be found."

Mattie, a few chairs down, overheard the conversation and yelled, "Marguerite spent one hundred fifty thousand dollars on a Mexican kidney a few months back."

The patients in the unit who heard that tidbit gaped at Mattie, jaws dropping.

J.R. wondered aloud if a Mexican kidney would suddenly give Marguerite a taste for tacos and Tequila. "Can you picture her dancing through the unit with maracas?"

Everyone laughed at the idea.

Mr. Freeman said, "It's a funny thought, but maybe not so far-fetched. I heard of a person who had a heart transplant from someone who loved baseball. Baseball bored her before the transplant, but afterwards it became her obsession. Another person started loving classical music after receiving a heart from a violinist. A gay person became straight after receiving a heart from a straight person."

At that point, a loud voice boomed from the lobby. "I'm here to check on my son." Darnell sank a little in his chair. "That's Mama. Brace yourselves."

J.R. grinned. "So now I'll get my chance to meet a *real* battle-axe."

Darnell shot him a pleading look. "Please, whatever you do, don't let her know I called her that."

Rachel turned to see a woman in her sixties with steel wool hair and the most beautiful green eyes she had ever seen. She wore a bright African patterned dress and scarf around her head.

Rachel greeted her. "Can I help you?"

"I'm Darnell's Mama." She strode past her into the unit.

Rachel stopped her. "We have a visitor protocol. You need to wash your hands and put on a gown." Rachel assisted her in putting a gown on that barely covered her substantial body. She found a chair for her to sit next to Darnell. Rachel returned to her work, watching Darnell's Mama out of the corner of her eye.

Mama sat on the little chair, but her presence filled the entire dialysis unit.

Darnell asked, "Mama, what brings you here? Is every-thing okay?"

"No, everything be fine. After you lost all your blood here, I wanted to be sure they was takin' good care of you." She glanced around the unit.

"Mama, I want you to meet J.R. on my left and Mr. Freeman on my right. J.R. is the one who saved my life that day."

Mr. Freeman interjected, "I would have saved his life too. J.R. just has the bigger mouth. We all love Darnell. You have done a great job of raising such a fine young man."

"It's not easy raising kids these days. Too many guns and drugs and not enough food and books. Not all my kids turned out like Darnell. I keep praying though."

Mr. Freeman nodded. "I know. I grew up in the hood. It's not easy."

J.R. squinted and took a good look at Mama. "You look so familiar, like I know you from somewhere."

"I just look familiar because I look like Aunt Jemima on the pancake boxes."

J.R. tilted his head, "Is that you, Ruby?"

She turned, took a good look at him and grinned. "Elijah! I haven't seen ya since high school." She jumped out of her chair and gave him a big hug and kissed his cheek.

"Oh, now you'll kiss me, forty years too late. You had to go and marry Slick Willie." He touched her cheek ever so gently with his free hand.

"Yeah, he was slick, but he was a good man. We only had a few years together. He died at twenty-three with bad kidneys. They didn't dialyze black people those days. We had one daughter, Jasmine. She had three babies; Shanita is the oldest, Darnell the middle one, and Will the youngest. Jasmine died giving birth to Will. She had 'pressure' and something wrong with her kidneys. I never knew what it was that killed her. I raised her children like my own."

She looked intently at J.R. "Do you remember those walks through Liberty Boulevard Park? You made me laugh no matter what was going on, even during the riots you found something to joke about."

J.R. just kept smiling. "Ruby, Ruby, Ruby, I can't believe it's really you…"

- Chapter 17 -

It was a gray day with the wind howling around the building and Lake Erie's waves crashing the shore. Darnell loved practicing his guitar when it was noisy outside. He could belt out his songs, and no one would complain about his off-key singing and tell him to get his voice tuned. He was singing at the top of his lungs when his younger brother Will walked onto the balcony. Will and Darnell could pass for twins. They were the same height and build, both had dreadlocks and hazel eyes. "Bad idea to leave your apartment door wide open in this neighborhood. I locked it when I came in."

Darnell's face widened into a big smile. "I haven't seen you in months. It's good to see you." He stood and gave his brother a hug.

Will sat on the other balcony chair and took a deep breath. "The cops are after me. They busted the club last night. We scattered. They chased me down a few streets and alleys and shit, until they gave up. I never knew high school hoops would come in so handy. I need to lay low for a few days. Can I stay here until things cool off?" He leaned back on the chair next to Darnell, looking at him intently.

Darnell was quiet for several long minutes as he watched the waves. He loved his brother dearly and enjoyed his company, but hated the drugs and trouble that accompanied him everywhere.

"I suppose you could sleep on what's left of Mama's lumpy couch. We may have jumped on it too many times when we were kids. One rule though; you can't bring drugs or your drug buddies here. The transplant office checks my blood monthly for drugs. Even being around someone smoking weed will show up in my blood."

"Shit, you been waiting for a transplant forever."

"Yeah, waiting for the right young person to die suddenly. Car accidents are nice, gunshot wounds also convenient."

Will shook his head. "Can't imagine waiting for someone to die so you can have their kidney. Some poor family is going to be full of grief for your chance at life off dialysis."

Darnell nodded. "I try not to think about that part."

Will then said, "Maybe I can give you one of my kidneys. The party enders wouldn't think of looking for me in the hospital."

"You're thinking of giving me a kidney?"

"I'm getting tired of you be doing dialysis day in and day out, year in and year out. What do I need to do?"

"I don't know all the details. I know it takes a few months of testing, like making sure you haven't contracted any diseases in your profession that you could donate along with your kidney. They also want to be sure I'm not coercing you in any way."

Will sighed. "I suppose I'll have to tell them the truth. You've been coercing me into everything my whole life. In addition to beating me up daily, you made me do my fucking homework, you forced me to play hoops, now you're coercing me to give you one of my kidneys."

"I wish I could coerce you to stop doing drugs. Why are you doing the same shit that got you the first prison term?"

He grinned. "I have an honorable profession as a drug rep."

Darnell frowned. "Not funny. I'm worried about you. I've started praying for you like Mama."

Will jabbed his arm playfully. "That's pathetic. Now I'm worried about you." He turned serious. "I've tried to find other ways to make money, but who is going to hire a black man with a felony and no marketable skills except selling drugs?

I tried bro. The best job I could get was flipping burgers at McDonalds, and they pay shit."

"Keep looking, you'll find something. You have people smarts. When you were younger everyone said that you could sell sunscreen to a black man living in the Arctic Circle."

"It's hard to get out of this business. People have things on me. Can I borrow your gun since you're not a security guard anymore? For self-protection."

"I sold it to a gun dealer when I lost the job. I didn't want to have a gun in my apartment with Shanita's boys wandering around getting into every nook and cranny."

"I haven't seen her, nor those two little scrappers, for the longest time. Maybe I'll visit them today."

"You'll have to wait until after supper. Shanita picks up Clarence and Lester from daycare after work around five. They eat around six, and the bedtime ritual starts at seven-thirty. Maybe we can help Shanita with baths and bedtime stories tonight. You're not allowed to rile them up at bedtime though, or Shanita will whip you. Sometimes I give them a day off from daycare to play with them. Maybe we can take them fishing on my day off from dialysis, the day after tomorrow. I've been promising to take them fishing all summer.

Will nodded. "I'd like that."

"I could use your help. They're a handful. They remind me of the two of us when we were little, wrestling together like little bear cubs. By the way, Mama is dating J.R., the man who sits next to me in dialysis. J.R. drives her anywhere she wants. She doesn't need or want me to drive her around anymore. They've only been together a few weeks and already talking of marriage."

"Marriage? Did you try to talk her out of it? I can't picture Mama with a man."

"Tell me about it. Of course I tried. Apparently, they knew each other in high school. J.R. says life is short and he's been waiting for her for her for forty years. Mama just smiles and dotes over him."

The two brothers wandered to the refrigerator to get some beer.

Will noticed the art history book open on the kitchen table and picked it up.

"What's this?"

"The only good thing about being on dialysis is that the Bureau of Vocational Rehab will pay my college tuition."

"I know you don't think of yourself as lucky, being on dialysis and all, but at least you have a future."

Darnell didn't feel lucky and couldn't envision a future for his life, so he changed the subject. "How's your love life? Are you still with Lanetta?"

"When I was in prison, she be writing me letters, visiting me, telling me she loved me all mushy and then when I got out, I discovered that she been seeing Jimmy the whole time. I hear they now have a kid."

"Lousy two-timer. My love life is worse than yours though. I'm in love with one of my nurses, but I don't have a chance with her. Being a dialysis patient is a turnoff for attracting babes."

They heard a pounding on the door, looked at each other, and panicked.

Darnell whispered hoarsely, "Sounds like the cops found you already." He pointed to a corner on the balcony. "Hide there. You can't see it from my apartment, nor can you see it from outside. Take your beer with you."

Darnell sauntered slowly to the door, a can of beer in his hand. He opened the door slowly, saw two cops, and asked politely, "Can I help you?"

They attacked Darnell; one of them grabbed his dread-locks and smashed his head against the door jamb. There was a loud crack and he fell to the ground. The beer can fell out of his hands, spilling onto the floor. They flipped him over, pinned his arms behind him, and applied handcuffs.

He moaned. "Those handcuffs are too tight; they're hurting my dialysis fistula." At that request, one cop stood and used his foot to press Darnell's arm tighter against his back. They started kicking him. Darnell cried out.

Will heard the commotion and rushed from his hiding place on the balcony. He placed his beer on the counter and held his arms out to be handcuffed. "I'm the one you're looking for. Leave my brother alone. He be a dialysis patient. He knows nothing about what I do."

They did a double take on seeing Will looking so much like Darnell. "We're arresting you both. Your brother was harboring a fugitive, and you fled the scene of a crime last night."

The other cop put handcuffs on Will and nodded towards Darnell. "It'd be too much trouble to bring that one in. We'd have to waste officers' time guarding him during dialysis sessions."

The cop released his foot from Darnell's back, knelt, and unlocked Darnell's handcuffs. Darnell turned his head and made eye contact with Will.

Will, distressed, shook his head and mouthed, "I'm sorry, Bro."

The cop that released the handcuffs on Darnell said, "You need to clean this shithole apartment," as he kicked the beer can. It rolled away, spilling a tiny river of beer. He followed his partner as they escorted Will out of the apartment.

After they left, Darnell rolled to his back and lay on the floor, trying to gather his wits about him. Everything hurt. He moaned and wondered if he was dying. After a while he gingerly pushed himself to a seated position with an excruciating headache, a sore back, painful ribs, and a throbbing fistula. He thought of Will and the implications of his arrest. He touched his fingers to his fistula to check the pulse and vibration to make sure it still worked but couldn't find either. "Fuck!" He started crying.

- Chapter 18 -

The following morning, Darnell called the dialysis unit to tell them that his fistula had stopped working. Rachel instructed him to come in anyway. If they couldn't use it for dialysis, she would call the vascular surgeon on call and arrange to get it de-clotted.

A few hours later Darnell hobbled into the unit, leaning to his left side with a misshapen head. He held on to a large stick to help him stand straight. His right eye was discolored and swollen shut.

Rachel saw him limping in pain with his disfigured face, and her gut twisted. She ran to him and helped him sit in the waiting room. "Oh my God! What happened to you?"

His voice was weak and gravelly as he told Rachel the story.

Rachel examined his red and swollen fistula arm. She held his arm tenderly as she searched for any pulse or vibration, hoping that they could still use it for dialysis. She took her stethoscope and listened before shaking her head. "You're right. It is clotted off. I'm sorry."

She still had her hand on his arm when she touched his head and felt the protruding lump where his head had smashed against the door jamb. "I'm calling an ambulance. I can't believe the cops beat you up like this." She asked the secretary to dial 911 and get the papers from his chart together.

"I don't want your sympathy or anyone's sympathy. When my brother told the cops I was a dialysis patient, they released me. Their disdain hurt more than the beating. I wish I could have roughed them up a bit."

"Maybe you can rough them up in court. I'm not sending you to the ER for sympathy. Your injuries need to be documented."

He looked at her sideways. "I don't have the money to take them to court."

Rachel said, "There is a Free Legal Aid Society in Cleveland. They might help. Let me ask my fiancé, who is a lawyer, for his opinion."

"You're engaged? Where's your engagement ring?"

"I didn't want a diamond after seeing the movie, Blood Diamond."

A siren squealed in the distance, and soon flashing lights indicated the ambulance had arrived. When the paramedics walked in, rolling the stretcher, Darnell frowned, stood up gingerly, and told them he could walk.

A few hours later, Rachel called the ER to learn that Darnell was being admitted. He had a cracked skull and two broken ribs. The fistula was not repairable, so the vascular surgeon had the radiologist put a permanent catheter in Darnell's chest so he could receive dialysis before he took him to surgery to create a new fistula. The catheter would remain in his chest for the few months it takes for a new fistula to mature.

———————

That evening, as they ate dinner, Rachel told Steve what had happened to Darnell, and the injuries he sustained as a result.

Steve was interested. "He may be able to sue the cops for police brutality."

"His only source of income is disability."

"Let me discuss it with my partners. I'd like to take his case on a contingency basis. He pays me only if I get a favorable settlement. The story of police beating a vulnerable dialysis patient would hit the news for sure and bring publicity to our firm. It may help me build my clientele."

Rachel smiled, walked around the table, sat on Steve's lap, and gave him a big hug. "That would be awesome!"

- Chapter 19 -

Elizabeth took a week off work after Ebony's death. As she mourned, she spent the week eliminating the evidence of Ebony's sojourn with her family. She gave away Ebony's dog bowls, dog bed, brushes, leashes, nail clippers, and toys. She spent hours vacuuming dog fur out of carpets and Ebony's blue chair. Ebony's fur had even found its way into her refrigerator.

The day she returned to work she battled weariness and fatigue as she glanced around the unit. It was the day to review patients' monthly labs. The patients looked unusually sick and needy, and the day ahead overwhelmed her. She reviewed the first patient's labs with him and recommended some needed dietary changes, and he flipped out. He called Elizabeth a bitch and told her that she had no idea how difficult it was coming to dialysis day in and day out and following the stupid dialysis diet.

Elizabeth moved on to the next patient, but not before saying, "I understand more than you think I do." As Elizabeth rounded, she heard Rachel kidding J.R. about leaving a cup of wine for him at Passover. The patients around him were laughing. Elizabeth wandered over, hoping for a good laugh.

"What's so funny?"

"I'd like you to meet Elijah James Richards. All this time we thought his name was just J.R....but last Monday, when Darnell's mom came to see the unit, she told us his name is really Elijah.

J.R. groaned, "That is exactly why I'm J.R. I didn't want anyone expecting me to perform miracles in the dialysis unit. Too much responsibility."

After a few minutes of small talk, Rachel and Elizabeth walked to the nurse's station as Rachel updated Elizabeth on the happenings in the unit the past week. "Darnell got beaten up by the police. Apparently, they thought he was his brother. They ruined his fistula and cracked his skull. He is in the hospital now. Dr. Brady finally got that transplant from his brother, so far, it's working well. We're all hoping he takes better care of it than he took care of his diabetes. Marguerite has been AWOL for two months now. A new patient will be starting in her chair tomorrow. Can you review the chart and write orders? Harriet is back from the hospital and has decided to stop dialysis."

Elizabeth stopped walking, "What??"

"You'll see. She has an invitation for you."

When Elizabeth arrived at Harriet's chair, the petite, wrinkled schoolteacher, the mother of the corner pod, she handed her a colorful invitation to her going away party the coming Saturday.

"Where are you going?"

"Today is my last dialysis. I'm done. I just came today to pass out invitations. I might not stay for the whole treatment. I'll sign one of those 'leaving against medical advice forms' one last time just for the hell of it."

"If you stop dialysis, you'll die."

"I know. I'm dying. That last hospitalization did me in. I can't take care of myself anymore."

"But you're young, only fifty-nine."

"My body is three hundred years old."

"You can do physical therapy to regain your strength. Don't you still have children to raise or grandchildren to spoil?"

"No grandkids yet, but my daughters are grown and living on their own. I've spent the past twenty-five years raising them as a single mom, working full-time while doing dialysis or trying to keep a transplanted kidney alive. This past year I've suffered two broken bones, a heart attack, a blood infection, and heart failure three times. I spent more time in the hospital or rehab than at home. I see the writing on the wall. It is not just my kidneys; my entire body is failing. It's time to turn off the lights and shut the door."

"You could try for another kidney transplant," Elizabeth offered hopefully.

"No, even *if* the transplant team considered me healthy enough for a transplant, I wouldn't consider it. There are three dead kidneys floating in my body already."

"What do your daughters have to say about all this?"

"They cried, but overall, they're supportive. They'll take turns staying with me day and night until I pass."

"Are you sure you aren't just depressed? Perhaps you'd like to see a psychiatrist first?"

"You sound like Dr. Burnouf."

Elizabeth nodded. "Yeah, guess I do. I've worked with him for so many years that I probably *am* starting to sound like him. Did you invite him to the party?"

"He wouldn't even make a hospice referral for me. Until this point, he's always been there for me, finding me one more chance at life. I guess he can't handle the thought of letting me go."

"Your death is going to be difficult for a lot of people, including me." Elizabeth asked, "Is everyone in the corner pod coming?"

"Some of them are angry, thinking that what I am doing is a sin. Robert's been talking to them. Maybe they'll change their minds by Saturday. I am hoping to see everyone one last time."

"It is hard to think of just seeing you one last time. This unit won't be the same without you. Even when you were sick or not feeling well, you inspired us all."

Elizabeth fingered the invitation, really looking at it now. A quote at the top said, *Death isn't extinguishing the light: it's putting out the lamp because dawn has come*, by Rabindranath Tagore. She hadn't heard of this Rabindranath person but liked the quote instantly. Elizabeth thought that perhaps this party might be the perfect opportunity to broach the subject of her own choice not to start dialysis with her daughters. She fumbled some more with the invitation and asked tentatively if she could bring her daughters to the party.

"Well, I don't know them, but I suppose it would be okay… Why in the world would you want to bring them?"

"I have kidney disease, late Stage four from diabetes, and have chosen to forgo dialysis. I want to prepare my daughters for my decision."

Harriet looked surprised and said in a loud voice, "Coward! Aren't you even going to give it a try? Trust me, it's not as bad as it looks. Dialysis gave me a chance at life, a chance to raise my children, a chance to continue loving the people in my life. Eli, I respect your judgment in so many ways, but that's a horrible decision."

Elizabeth was caught off guard by Harriet's response. She had hoped to find an ally, a co-conspirator in Harriet. She flustered as she slipped the invitation into her pocket. "On second thought, I don't think I'll be bringing my daughters."

Harriet smiled kindly at her and nodded. Elizabeth moved to the next patient, Howard the pawnbroker, who frequently skipped his treatments or cut them short.

He shook his head, "I can't imagine coming to dialysis and not having her in that chair. It won't be the same without her."

"That's how we feel when you skip your treatments, Howard. One of these days, skipping dialysis is going to kill you, and someone else will be sitting in your chair." He looked away and pretended not to hear as Elizabeth berated herself. *I'm planning on skipping dialysis altogether. I'm such a hypocrite.*

- Chapter 20 -

Later that morning the unit secretary handed Rachel a letter. It had the United Dialysis Associates letterhead on the envelope. Rachel's stomach dropped to the floor. She had been waiting for this letter and not waiting at the same time. Somehow as the weeks went by, she had been able to block the looming decision from her consciousness; day-to-day life had resumed its rhythm. The envelope reminded her of her uncertain future, so she shoved it into her pocket without reading it. Rachel completed the first shift medications and found Elizabeth. "Eli, I need to talk with you. Can I treat you to lunch today?"

They chose the same picnic table where they had eaten lunch in May. It was now the beginning of September. The days were still warm, but the light was muted and the shadows longer. Clouds occasionally covered the sun, lending a chill to the air. A few precocious leaves released their grasp on the branches and floated on the breeze until they scraped the pavement.

Once their napkins and drinks were situated for the picnic, Rachel started explaining. "I'm sure you heard I let Ethel die in the unit without starting CPR."

"No secrets in a dialysis unit. I figured there was another side to the story, and you would tell me eventually.

Rachel told her everything about Ethel's death, and subsequent investigation. She told Elizabeth how she's been waiting on pins and needles for the verdict, looking at want-ads, and considering returning to school to become a librarian.

She reached into her pocket and pulled out the official-looking envelope. "This came today." She shoved the envelope towards Elizabeth.

"You didn't open it?"

“Afraid to. Afraid I may need resuscitation.”

“So…you want me to open it?”

“Please.”

Elizabeth opened it slowly with a concerned look on her face and, as she read the letter, broke into a grin. She pushed the opened letter back to Rachel.

Mr. Peter Swanson, CCHT
Regional Chief of Dialysis
United Dialysis Associates
Cleveland, Ohio

August 28, 2019

Dear Ms. Rachel Rosen RN,

I am writing this letter to inform you that we identified the problem with machine #twenty-three. A glitch in the computer software shuts down the venous pressure alarm when it should be activated. Similar situations have occurred in other units, but you are the one who recognized the pattern.

We reported the problem to the manufacturer and are in the process of removing all the new Emerson machines from our dialysis units. They are working on a software fix, but it may result in the recall of all the Emerson dialysis machines manufactured in the past two years.

Thank you for bringing this to our attention. I am going to ask the regional vice president to give you special recognition at our next quarterly meeting.

I have also sent a copy of this letter to your dialysis unit manager, Ms. Leggett.

Sincerely,
Peter Swanson CCHT
Regional Chief of Dialysis

"It sounds like good news, but what exactly is this about?"

She told her the story of machine number twenty-three.

"Rachel, you may have saved several lives not just in our unit but other units."

"I still have the conclusion of the internal investigation hanging over my head."

Elizabeth shook her head, "It doesn't make sense. If they were going to fire you, or report you to the Board of Nursing, you'd have been gone weeks ago."

Rachel nodded. "I hope you're right. It's the not knowing that gnaws on me."

Rachel changed the subject. "Are you going to Harriet's going away party?"

"I wouldn't miss it for the world."

"Really? Why?"

"Patients have withdrawn from dialysis, but Harriet is the first I've known of to give herself a going away party. I want to see how she pulls it off. We all die, but we usually don't have control over the when or how. Harriet is planning the circumstances of her death. During her last hospitalization she was on the ventilator for three weeks. I suspect she wants to spare her children the agonizing decision of turning off the ventilator the next time."

"Do you think I'll be crossing boundaries by going?"

"Of course."

"Will you go with me? I don't expect Steve to want to come."

"I don't relish going alone either. Perhaps afterwards we can stop for a glass of wine and discuss everything."

Rachel nodded, "I bet we'll be needing a glass of wine afterwards."

- Chapter 21 -

Rachel stopped by the pier after work to think about the letter and Harriet's going away party, but mainly to watch the waves and sun glinting on the water. She had only a few minutes to spare. Steve's work cocktail party was that evening. She hated cocktail parties; in addition to being bored to tears, cocktail dresses made her feel like a Barbie doll toy.

Lake Erie was blue and glad and caressed all those on its shore with a gentle breeze. The water gently rolled and tumbled with sailboats gliding in the distance. She liked this pier because there was a canopy covering a few benches. She could be close to the water and still be in the shade.

She watched the couples milling around and wondered about her and Steve. She felt lonely around him. Some days she didn't even like him. She excused his behavior, thinking that perhaps the pressure of working to be a partner in his firm was making him irritable. She wondered if they were going through an ordinary rough patch in their relationship or if it was time to back out of the wedding. She didn't know if she had the guts to call the wedding off.

She watched the people strolling the pier. An elderly couple walked slowly together; their heads close in conversation. The woman had a limp, and her companion was careful to watch her steps and support her arm as they walked. She wondered if Steve would be as careful supporting her steps if she were old and limping. Then she observed another couple, the man rode an electric scooter, his companion was obese with a bright orange sleeveless top that accentuated the rolls of love handles up and down the sides of her torso. Her pink bra straps clashed with the orange top and made grooves in her shoulders. Frizzy maroon hair completed the portrait. Rachel gawked for a moment. *They seem to be enjoying each other's company though. Her looks and outfit didn't seem to bother him.*

She needed to get home to get ready for the cocktail party but didn't want to leave quite yet. She let her gaze wander for just a few more moments, taking in all the people hanging around the pier. On the right side of the pier, close to the end, she noticed three figures: a black man with a fishing rod and on each side of him a tiny figure with a tiny fishing rod. *That can't be Darnell. He's supposed to be in the hospital.* She sauntered over to get a closer look. As she approached, she saw the dressing from the surgery on his right arm and knew it was him. The two little boys on each side snuggled close and were talking and laughing as they swung their legs back and forth in the open air below the pier. She suddenly felt shy and turned to walk away, but Darnell saw her, and a big grin exploded on his face. She winced at his misshapen face and black eye.

"Darnell, you're supposed to be in the hospital."

"I signed out AMA this morning. I didn't want to miss the sun and the breeze today. Seeing this day from the window of my hospital room would hurt more than my broken ribs. Besides, I've been promising my nephews I'd take them fishing for weeks."

Both little boys looked at Darnell and snuggled a little closer.

"How are you feeling?"

"Let's see…my ribs are sore, my arm is sore, and my head hurts. The most brutal pain, though, is that the surgery for my new fistula disfigured the tattoo of the beautiful lady on my right arm. She lost a boob, half a head of hair, an arm, and a leg."

Rachel laughed. "Maybe they'll grow back. I hope they took a picture of your face in the hospital."

"They took a lot of x-rays and a CT scan, but no one took a regular picture."

Rachel whipped out her phone and asked if he minded if she took a picture of him. Then she had second thoughts because of HIPAA laws. "Can I use your phone so you can have the picture?"

He handed it to her, "Good idea. I don't want you having any ugly pictures of me in your phone."

Rachel took several pictures of his face, trying to find the best angle, the best lighting, while keeping the little boys out of the picture. "These pictures may help your court case. My fiancé Steve told me he would take your case on a contingency basis, meaning no money out of your pocket up front, but if he wins your case, he gets one-third of the settlement. His name is Steve Silverman; I put his number in your phone. Give him a phone call early next week."

By this time, the twins wanted to get rid of Rachel, the intruder on their time with their uncle. "Go away!" both boys said in unison.

Rachel turned to leave. "Sorry to bother your fishing."

"Nah, don't go yet," coaxed Darnell. "Sit for just a few minutes. There won't be many more days like today."

Rachel sat down on the pier a few feet away from one of the little boys and smiled.

"These are my two nephews, Clarence and Lester." He patted each one on the head as he said their names. "Show your manners and say 'Hi' to Rachel. She is my nurse sometimes when I have dialysis." They both mumbled "Hi," and turned and snuggled closer to Darnell. Darnell smiled and hugged them both. "They're not usually this shy."

Rachel smiled, "Nice to meet you Clarence and Lester." She wanted to ruffle their little dreadlocks but knew that impulse wouldn't be welcomed.

"I'm teaching my nephews how to fish. I was just telling them that a good fisherman always needs to keep his hook in the water, waiting for opportunities. When you least expect it, a great big fish might come sauntering by."

Rachel said, "I think it's cool that J.R., I mean Elijah, and your Mama knew each other in high school."

He scrunched his face and raised his eyebrows, looking even more grotesque. He said in a low voice, "When I got out of the hospital today, I stopped by Mama's, and she was sitting on the front porch with J.R., the two of them yakking away. J.R. told me how wild and beautiful Mama used to be with her afro and lithe body. They climbed trees together in Liberty Park. I've only known her as Mama, never imagining her any other way. Intellectually, I knew she was young once, maybe beautiful, but somehow…" He shook his head, "I still can't picture her climbing a tree."

"That same thing happens to me when I care for dialysis patients. I have a hard time imagining that they were once different and had lives before dialysis. I get this frozen idea in my mind that they were always like they are now, half alive, gray, crotchety, and sick. I forget that they were once young and beautiful."

He frowned as he looked into her eyes. "Is that how you think of me? Half alive? Do I seem sickly to you?"

"Oh God, no. I shouldn't have said that. I'm an idiot. You are handsome and alive…but today, your face is kind of ugly…"

By this time, Clarence and Lester, bored with fishing, had started rummaging through Darnell's tackle box.

"Hey, you two, that box is off limits. There are sharp hooks in there. Let's put the fishing tackle away and throw stones in the water from the shore." The two boys forgot their shyness and started chasing each other around the pier. Darnell gingerly reached out, grabbed them both and showed them the water. "You can't run on this pier; if you fall off, the lake will swallow you up. What was I thinking? I better give you swimming lessons before I give you more fishing lessons."

Rachel saw him wince when he caught his nephews. "Let me gather the fishing tackle while you hang on to your nephews." She picked up two little rods and one big rod and noticed that each of them had colorful bobbers and weights, but none of them had fishing hooks or bait on them. She shook her head, "I guess you weren't really expecting to catch fish today."

"I know these guys. I wasn't going to risk a fishhook in one of their eyes. I knew this fishing excursion wouldn't last more than a few minutes. Their attention span is about twenty seconds. I was impressed that they sat patiently with me for so long. I did catch a fish today though."

"Where is it? Your bucket's empty."

"The fish I caught today is too big for a bucket." He quickly turned his attention to his nephews. "Clarence and Lester, hold on to each other's hands." He took the fishing rods and tackle from Rachel and instructed her to hold on to Clarence's hand while he held on to Lester's. She smiled as Clarence put his little hand into hers without question or complaint.

The foursome sauntered up the pier to the shore, holding hands.

A passerby shook his head in disapproval and said to Darnell, "Stick with your own kind kid. That woman is forbidden fruit."

Rachel glanced at Darnell, wondering how he would respond. He ignored the comment, remaining cool and collected.

Rachel turned and yelled at the man's back as he walked away, "You're an imbecile if you think skin color matters more than what's in a person's heart!" As soon as she said it, she knew her outburst wasn't helpful. She looked at Darnell and saw the faintest wisp of a smile cross his bruised and swollen face. Not knowing how to redeem her outburst, she asked,

"Hey, are you going to Harriet's going away party?"

"Harriet asked me to play the guitar and sing Gospel hymns. Not my usual repertoire. I haven't practiced since I got beat up. I may be too sore to play anything, and my singing might come out as a long, low moan."

"Be sure to take some pain medication before you play."

Darnell said, "I think the party is going to be weird though. Kind of like a funeral with the dead person sitting upright in the casket and looking around. Are you coming?"

After hearing he was going to be there, she knew she would attend but said, "I don't know, there are certain professional boundaries to observe as a nurse."

"Fuck boundaries. This is about life and death."

When they arrived at the shore, Rachel let go of Clarence's hand. "I gotta run. I'm late for a cocktail party." She squatted down to Clarence and Lester and asked them for a hug, and they both hugged her. "Nice to meet you guys." She ran up the path to the parking lot and hopped in her car.

- Chapter 22 -

Rachel sped on the freeway on her way home. She was late again and knew Steve would be upset. Her stomach churned. She berated herself for stopping at the lake after work. She wondered if she was being passive-aggressive because a stupid cocktail party was the last place she wanted to be. She also ruminated over the fact that she always went to places he wanted to go, but Steve never came with her to events she wanted to go to.

She pulled into her driveway, leapt out of her car, and ran into the house. "Hi Steve, sorry I'm late."

He met her at the door, fully dressed in suit and necktie. "Where have you been? We're an hour late already. By the time you get yourself all prettied up we'll be two hours late!"

"I can get ready in ten minutes. Sit on the couch and watch some baseball."

She ran into their bedroom, ripped off her scrubs, and put the cocktail dress on. It wouldn't zip up though. "Shit, I must have gained weight since the last time I wore this. It's all those snacks and lunches that patients' families bring in." She rifled through her closet, looking for something else to wear. She put on a sensible skirt and top, looked in the mirror and realized she looked like a schoolmarm. She didn't have time to try other outfits though and ran down the stairs.

She ran into the living room and announced, "I'm ready."

He saw her outfit, frowned, and asked, "Where is that lovely cocktail dress that you have?"

"I couldn't get it zipped," she said sheepishly.

"You look like a librarian, not someone going to a cocktail party."

"Let's go. No one will notice or remember what I wore tonight."

"Why don't you care what you look like? This is important!"

"What is so important about it? I hope no promotion of yours depends upon what I wear to a cocktail party. I'm hungry. I hope they have some good hors d'oeuvres."

He groaned and walked past her to the car. As Steve drove, he lectured her ad nauseam on the importance of the corporate cocktail party as an opportunity to network and build relationships.

As he pontificated, Rachel stared out the window at the stoplights and houses going by. *Blah, blah, blah. I don't remember signing up to be his arm candy.*

When they arrived at the country club, Rachel and Steve exchanged pleasantries with his partners. After a few moments, Steve ditched her to go hobnob with his co-workers. Rachel, already bored with the need to act interested and interesting, found the bar, the hors d'oeuvres table, and noticed at the end of the room a covered veranda facing west, overlooking a golf course. There were couches on the veranda. It was a warm early autumn evening, and Rachel thought, *All is not lost. I can sit on the veranda, eat some food, drink some wine, and watch the sunset.* She ambled to the hors d'oeuvres table and piled her plate with shrimp, bacon-wrapped chestnuts, stuffed mushrooms, little cheese quiches, and mascarpone figs, not caring about the effect the appetizers would have on her ability to get into that cocktail dress next cocktail party. She knew Steve would be critical of her non-Kosher food choices and wondered if that's how her dialysis patients feel when they sneak forbidden foods. She meandered to the veranda to sit on a couch. She found one perfectly angled so she could watch the party and the sunset simultaneously. "Ahhh!" She was tired from the long day at work and rested her feet on the table in front of the couch.

She watched Steve suck up to his superiors and…and…

and…she squinted her eyes, was he flirting with that secretary? Their heads were close, and they gazed into each other's eyes, smiling. Their lips were close enough to kiss, and then he caressed her butt! The secretary sported a sexy cocktail dress that accentuated the curves in her body. Rachel couldn't remember the last time he touched her butt like that.

While she processed Steve's behavior with the secretary, one of Steve's partners sat down beside her. "Hello Rachel, do you remember me? I'm Anthony, an associate with Steve on the partner treadmill."

Rachel sat up straight, taking her feet off the table. "I remember your face, but I'm glad you reminded me of your name." She remembered him as the most handsome of Steve's associates with olive-colored skin, shiny black hair, blue eyes, and a nice smile. He had a presence about him.

"I hoped you'd be here tonight. At the last cocktail party, you told me that you work as a nurse in dialysis. My dad started dialysis three weeks ago and is miserable. He complains that dialysis turns him into a zombie. He acts like a zombie too. He sits all day in front of the TV, sometimes crying. I've never seen him cry before. I don't know what to do. I called my dad's doctor, and he told me that my dad's doing well on dialysis, very stable, and they are removing some of the extra fluid he gained over the past year. What do you think is going on?"

"I can't say for sure, but it sounds like he's grieving the loss of his kidneys. Most people ignore their kidneys until they're gone. What does your dad do for a living?"

"He's an electrician but hasn't been able to work because of his dialysis schedule, and I don't think he feels well enough to work these days anyway. My parents don't know what they're going to do without his income. They are worried about hospital bills and the possibility of losing his medical insurance."

Rachel nodded. "Lots of losses to mourn. The unit social worker can help him with his bills and insurance coverage.

You can call the unit any time and ask to speak with her. Her name is Betty. Has he seen the dietitian yet?"

"He mentioned that. I guess that's another loss. He is Italian and can't eat his favorite foods anymore."

"What's his name? I wonder if he's the new patient in our unit."

"Joseph Fiorelli."

Rachel nodded. "Yes, I know him. I thought he was making a good adjustment to dialysis too. I didn't see that he was so depressed." She craned her neck behind Anthony to see what Steve was up to. He had walked away from the sex bomb secretary and was talking with other partners.

Anthony pursued his questions. "How long does it take for a person to adjust to dialysis?"

Rachel returned her gaze to Anthony. "Everyone is different, and the losses are different. An eighty-year-old person has a lot less to lose than a forty-year-old. The eighty-year-old is finished with his career, has probably dealt with many losses already in his life, and, quite frankly, doesn't have much left to lose. A younger person has their career, identity, income, health, and a future full of hopes and dreams to lose. Sometimes people on dialysis lose their partners because their partners can't handle the losses." Rachel ate the last mascarpone fig. "Most people do adjust though. It takes time, usually months, sometimes a year. Hopefully, your dad will make friends in the dialysis unit. Patients help each other cope. We often tell patients that while it is a difficult adjustment, they will eventually settle into a new normal."

"What can I do to help him?" Anthony probed.

"I don't know." She shrugged her shoulders. "Maybe just sit with him when he cries. Find something that he enjoys and take him and your mom out. Let him know you still love him and will be there for him. He'll learn that dialysis isn't the end of his life, just the start of a different one. Now that I know what's going on with him, I'll keep an eye on him."

Partygoers wandered to the veranda where Rachel and Anthony were sitting, possibly hoping for fresh air, or perhaps to enjoy the evening's sunset. Streaks of gold suffused the porch as the sun melted onto the green edge of the golf course. A few people clapped the minute the sun set, followed by a moment of silence, punctuated by the chirping of crickets and katydids. For an encore, the undulating waves of clouds overhead continued the evening's light show with streaks of pinks, blues, purples, and grays.

The murmur of conversation resumed, but Rachel was awestruck at the beauty in the sky and wondered how anyone could speak. After a few minutes she overheard one of the partners discussing the police brutality case concerning Darnell and stood to join the conversation. She described Darnell's cracked skull, broken ribs, and clotted dialysis fistula and the surgery he needed to create a new one. A few of the younger attorneys felt that this might be a very opportune time for such a case. Police brutality had been in the news lately, especially white-on-black. A story like this in the news would bring publicity to the firm. One young attorney offered that they could possibly get a quarter of a million for the patient.

A heated argument ensued. Others felt the case didn't have a chance. A gruff, gray-haired lawyer with bushy eyebrows insisted that the doctrine of 'qualified immunity,' which was initially designed to give policemen breathing room in dangerous crisis situations, had become an absolute shield for law enforcement officers to act with impunity. He called it a 'license to kill.' He said the doctrine of qualified immunity has been effective in police brutality lawsuits to throw out even the most horrific cases. He went on to say that it created a situation of 'heads the police win, tails the plaintiff loses.' He looked at Rachel, "Your patient would have a much better chance if he were white."

Rachel mumbled, "The assault wouldn't have happened if he were white."

Before she knew it, the party ended, and a river of people floated to their cars. Rachel got into the car with Steve and, as soon as she closed the passenger side door, she blurted out, "I saw you putting your hand on your secretary's butt. What is that about? Is there something between the two of you?"

"You're imagining things. Why are you always so paranoid? I saw you holding court on the veranda with all my partners. Is there anything between you and one of them?"

"No. I don't know them, nor do I work with them."

There was a deafening silence in the car for a few miles. Rachel felt Steve was lying to her but began to doubt herself, wondering if she saw what she thought she saw. "Tomorrow evening one of my patients is having a going away party. Will you come with me?"

"Where is she going?"

"Stopping dialysis. She plans to die."

"That sounds awful. Why do you want to go?"

"I love her and want to say goodbye."

"The Cleveland Indians are playing the Detroit Tigers tomorrow. If they win, they head to the playoffs. Simon and I are meeting at the Gangs Bar to watch it."

"I knew you wouldn't want to come with me. My backup plan is to go with Eli, the nurse practitioner I work with."

That night Rachel couldn't sleep. She tossed and turned as the clock ticked. She questioned herself again about seeing Steve put his hand on his secretary's butt and decided that she saw correctly. She could trust her eyes. She wondered if they were having an affair and if that woman (and not Simon) would be at the Gang's Bar tomorrow night.

She mulled over their relationship. They had met a lifetime ago in the same Bar Mitzvah class at the temple and spent many afternoons studying Hebrew together while playing footsie under the table. There was a time when they couldn't keep their hands off each other. She remembered longing for his touch and kisses – lately, not so much. She remembered their first kiss at his little sister's Bat Mitzvah party, slow dancing in the corner with the giant orb overhead scattering stars everywhere. She remembered the first time they had sex as seniors in high school, in a little picnic alcove at Mentor Headlands on Lake Erie. They were clumsy and fumbling but consumed with desire for each other. She remembered the hours after sex when they snuggled on a blanket watching the waves. Sand coated their skin, their hair, and all their body crevices. Steve was the only man she thought she would ever love.

What happened? Was it Steve or she that had changed? Perhaps the pressure to achieve partner was too much for him. She wondered if she was the problem with her insecurities as she navigated the roles and responsibilities of being a nurse. Her thoughts then veered back to his secretary. *Does he love her now? Are they having sex? Maybe he just doesn't love me anymore.* And then there was the other question nagging her heart: *Do I still love him?*

She also fretted about the senior law partner's comments that there was little chance for Darnell's case to be successful. When she first saw Darnell after the beating, she felt it was an open-and-shut case of unjustified police brutality. What the lawyer said at the party was disturbing. It didn't seem fair. She wanted Darnell to win this case. *I hope I didn't give him false hope.*

- Chapter 23 -

On the evening of Harriet's going away party, Rachel called Elizabeth to ask what time she was picking her up. "What do I wear to a going away party/funeral? Should I wear black? Should I wear a dress?"

Elizabeth replied, "I'm thinking casual. Remember that some of the guests will be people on dialysis who often don't have money for fancy clothes."

Rachel found a pair of nice slacks and a blouse. She also grabbed a light jacket to carry because the evenings were getting cooler. It had again taken her a few attempts to find a pair of slacks that would button up easily. She sat on the front stoop waiting for Eli and considered other symptoms she had been ignoring; her breasts were tender, and she was nauseous some mornings. *Maybe it wasn't the junk food...could I...could I...be pregnant?* She was on Seasonale, the birth control pill, where she had four periods a year, so she didn't pay attention to when her periods arrived or didn't. Occasionally, she skipped her period altogether.

Elizabeth arrived and they used GPS to find Harriet's house. Rachel asked Eli if she thought Harriet would be able to die comfortably after stopping dialysis. Elizabeth responded, "Harriet would need to avoid fluid. Too much fluid could end up in her lungs, making it difficult to breathe...but Harriet does a good job monitoring her fluid intake. I suspect she'll eat high potassium foods like chocolate, tomatoes, avocados, bananas, and potatoes. If she gets the potassium level high enough in her blood, she could probably slip away tonight with an abnormal heart rhythm as she sleeps."

Rachel listened to her prediction, puzzled at how Elizabeth had considered the matter in such detail.

Harriet lived in a tiny bungalow on a side street in Euclid. It was easy to find her house because of the balloons decorating the mailbox, the backyard outlined with white string lights, and a steady stream of people walking up her drive. Dusk came early, and the lights added a festive ambiance. Rachel and Elizabeth followed the guests to the backyard and joined the party.

Initially, Rachel stood on the sidelines and studied the gathering. She didn't know most of the people present but recognized a handful of patients. She saw various clusters of people who seemed to make up a cross-section of all the cultures and nationalities in Cleveland, including Asians, men wearing turbans, and women wearing hijabs. Children ran around playing. Rachel tried to guess how they knew Harriet. In her mind she sorted out the neighbors, friends, family, and former co-workers. Rachel recognized Harriet's four daughters as they had taken turns dropping their mom off and picking her up from dialysis. They were solemn and tearful. They tried to be good hostesses but appeared sad and huddled together. There was a low murmur of people talking and laughing. Rachel's heart skipped a beat when she heard Darnell in a dark corner playing softly on the guitar.

Then she spied Harriet, who looked like a little elf, dwarfed by her wheelchair. Her wheelchair was close to the wheelchair ramp at the rear of her house. She wore a green jacket with a dark blue blanket covering her legs. She was surrounded by well-wishers coming and going. As Elizabeth had predicted, Harriet had a box of Malley's chocolates on her lap. She would pick out a chocolate piece and pop it into her mouth as she spoke with the people surrounding her. When Rachel saw the chocolates, she tried to catch Elizabeth's eye, but she was busy talking with someone else.

As Rachel took the scene in, she saw Ms. Leggett holding court with several of the techs. Her stomach twisted. She grabbed Elizabeth's arm and whispered in her ear, "Shit! Ms. Leggett is here. I shouldn't have come."

Elizabeth grinned. "Well, in this context, Martha can't write you up for crossing boundaries or she'd have to write herself up too."

Rachel and Eli wandered to the food tables. There were two food tables well marked with large signs: a smaller table for dialysis patients and a larger one for everyone else. Rachel surveyed the dialysis table first. She saw a fruit salad consisting of pineapple, red grapes, and blueberries, a colorful arugula salad with peppers and radishes, a bowl of tabbouleh with pita bread for dipping, and cut-up carrots, celery, and cucumbers. She spied platters of cold salmon and warm chicken. Blueberry and apple pies were for dessert. Rachel felt touched that Harriet and her helpers had put so much thought into making the food safe and appetizing for her beloved friends. She noticed a few dialysis patients helping themselves to food choices from the regular table. J.R. blatantly disregarded the safe food table and piled his plate with the following items: fresh tomato salad, a cantaloupe melon salad, a hot dog, a hamburger slider with cheese, potato chips and two chocolate brownies for dessert. Every single food choice could either raise his blood pressure or make the potassium in his blood dangerously high!

She was aghast. *Oh, my God! He will be in the ER tonight for emergency dialysis.* She fought the urge to shake him or kick him. This was, after all, a party, and she didn't want to ruin it for anyone. However, she didn't succeed in restraining herself. She went to J.R. and asked him with a horrified look on her face, "Are you planning to die tonight along with Harriet?"

He smirked, tilted his head, and said, "I plan to go out styling."

Rachel watched him strut away, his lanky, bowlegged silhouette shaking with laughter. He set the plate before Ruby before glancing back at Rachel, still laughing.

Elizabeth, who had watched the scene, laughed. "Come on Rachel, tonight we forget we're nurses. We're not on the clock, nor are we responsible for anyone's decisions or behaviors but our own."

They filled their plates and sat at the only remaining seats in the yard at a picnic table across from Ruby and J.R. J.R. held the carrot he was munching like a cigar as he pontificated that he was blessed to be surrounded by the most beautiful women in the world on his final night on this earth. Rachel discretely gave J.R. the finger.

Ruby noticed and said to Rachel, "I'll kick him for ya," as she kicked his leg under the table.

He feigned injury but stopped his teasing. Ruby returned to her discussion with Howard, the pawn shop owner, to her right. She had a scheme that Darnell could pawn his motorcycle to raise enough bail money to get Will out of jail.

Rachel heard Darnell strumming his guitar in the corner and wondered what he thought of Mama's plan, and if he had the power to veto her. She glanced over at Darnell and realized he was already looking at her. Their eyes connected for a moment before Rachel turned her head away.

Toward the end of the meal, a gong sent shivers through the crowd. A quiet expectancy descended on the gathering. Darnell stopped playing guitar.

Robert, the retired pastor from the corner group, stood up to speak using a karaoke machine with a microphone. He prayed, "Lord we come together tonight to celebrate Harriet's life and to bless her as she continues her journey back to You, her creator and source of all life. Just as we're all destined to die sometime, we know her time is near. Her life was a glimmer of heaven for us. We pray for a peaceful, easy death. We are all afraid of dying, not knowing what awaits us on the other side." He cleared his throat. "We especially ask for your comfort and presence to be with all of us as we say our final goodbyes. Please comfort us in our grief when she is gone."

There were some scattered sobs and sniffles among the guests.

He then handed the microphone to Harriet.

She spoke in a quiet, quavering voice. "Dear Pastor Robert, my dialysis buddy and spiritual advisor for so many years, thank you for the prayer and blessings. I have one little correction to your prayer though. I'm not afraid to die. I have loved this life…all of it, including the pain and suffering. I know I'll love death as well. God has been with me in life and will be with me in death. I want to thank everyone for coming. It grieves me to say goodbye, but we all have to say goodbye sometime. My one dying request is that each of you says goodbye personally to me tonight before heading home."

J.R. got up to speak, taking the microphone from Harriet. "I've been to a lot of funerals where people tell stories and say kind words about the deceased. I've often wished the person could be a guest at their own funeral to hear the good things people say about them." He tilted his head. "Perhaps they do hear our words and stories?" He shrugged his shoulders. "I don't know. But tonight, we can make sure Harriet knows the difference her life has made in our lives. When I started dialysis ten years ago, I was scared and depressed, believing that I had reached the end of the line. I met Harriet in the waiting room, and she told me that she had been on dialysis for fifteen years so far. She told me to not be afraid, that dialysis was just a job she did to stay alive. She told me it was worth it." He bent towards Harriet, holding the microphone. "It has been worth it, and I want to thank you for being there for me those early months."

Neighbors told stories of raising their children together,

remembering backyard picnics and little scrapes their children cooked up. Once Harriet taught a young couple how to cook their first Thanksgiving turkey. They stuffed and dressed the turkey together before putting it in the oven. While the turkey roasted, Harriet invited the young couple to her house for drinks. While they toasted each other and shared Thanksgiving memories, Harriet's other neighbor traded the roasting turkey for a Cornish hen. When they returned to the house, Harriet urged the young husband to check the turkey. He opened the oven and shrieked, "The turkey shrank!"

A former student took the microphone and said that Harriet never let on that she had a dialysis life in addition to her teaching and motherhood life. She admitted that as students, they discussed the ropey veins on her arm, and missed her when she was hospitalized, but never considered her sick. The corner pod group stood up with Pastor Robert, arms on each other's shoulders and tears in their eyes. They told her they loved her and would talk about her when she was gone. Her four daughters got up and thanked her for being the best mother and father ever. Watching their mom deal with crisis after crisis had taught them to live one day at a time, putting one foot in front of the other.

Eventually people ran out of stories, and Harriet slouched to the side of her wheelchair, her head bobbing slightly. Pastor Robert took the microphone and, with authority, told people it was time to say goodbye, but before they did, Harriet requested that they sing some songs. He turned on the karaoke machine and led everyone in the yard in singing the 'Battle Hymn of the Republic,' 'Amazing Grace,' and 'When the Saints Go Marching In.'

Chills traveled up and down Rachel's spine with the music. She felt between worlds. She couldn't explain it. They sang a few more songs before people lined up in front of Harriet's wheelchair and Darnell resumed his guitar playing.

- Chapter 24 -

J.R. and Ruby left the table to mingle with friends from the dialysis unit. Rachel and Elizabeth saw the line and figured it would be a while before they got their turn to say goodbye. Rachel said, "She might not be afraid, but my stomach is full of butterflies. I could use a glass of wine; can I get one for you Eli?"

"Yes, I'd love a glass of white wine, and can you bring me another brownie please?" As Rachel walked back to the picnic table with the glasses of wine and the brownie, she saw Ms. Leggett sit across from Elizabeth at the spot J.R. and Ruby vacated. Rachel felt trapped. "Hi, Ms. Leggett," she said shyly, avoiding eye contact. "Can I get you a glass of wine or anything else?"

Ms. Leggett smiled. "Call me Martha. I've already had one glass of wine too many." Rachel had never seen Martha so genial and relaxed and had a fleeting notion to stock wine in Ms. Leggett's office. After she sat at the picnic table, Rachel took a large gulp from her own glass of wine, choked on it a bit, coughed, and sprayed some wine onto the table. Elizabeth and Martha didn't notice or at least pretended not to.

Elizabeth and Martha were discussing the party. Eli suggested that it was much better than dying in the ICU, intubated and unable to communicate. Martha argued that perhaps this party was too much for Harriet's daughters. A private family affair might have been better.

Eli countered that at least she saved her family the agonizing decision of turning off a ventilator. "You must admit, this beats a funeral. Many funeral attendees never get the chance to say goodbye.

The conversation veered to the too older nurses reminiscing about being young nurses together. They remembered past patients and laughed about some of the situations they had encountered. Rachel listened intently, trying to imagine them as younger versions of themselves. The evening air became chilly, and she put her jacket on.

Elizabeth asked Martha, "How did we live to be such old farts? Remember the days before gloves and surgical masks? I got blood, sputum, vomit, and feces on my hands daily; how did we survive? I can't imagine touching a patient these days without wearing gloves."

Martha shook her head. "So many changes over the years... where did the time go?"

Elizabeth leaned forward, elbows on the picnic table. "Do you remember slow codes?

When Rachel saw Martha nod, she asked, "What are slow codes?"

Eli looked at Rachel and explained, "Before the concept of DNR orders had been developed, we were required to resuscitate *everybody* even if their body was riddled with cancer and they were in pain with no hope of recovery. When nurses didn't want to increase the suffering of a dying patient they walked very slowly to the bedside and pretended to perform CPR; waiting to officially call for a code team when they were sure the patient had died."

Martha became agitated and raised her voice, "Why are you bringing that up now? You know I got written up and almost lost my license because of a slow code." She glanced at Rachel.

Elizabeth pushed Martha: "You remember how painful it was for you. Why would you put Rachel through the same torture?"

Martha put her head in her hands and shook her head. "I don't know. I don't know. I don't know."

Eli pushed even more: "Rachel has been walking on eggshells for weeks, expecting to lose her license any day, looking at want ads, considering different careers. You're not being fair to her. I suspect her position has been safe all along."

Martha looked at her hands folded on the table. "The investigators felt that you acted appropriately with the DNR order. There are no plans to fire you or report you to the Board of Nursing."

Rachel stood and walked away. She had no words. Her eyes filled with tears. She didn't realize until this moment how fearful she had been of losing her license.

She wandered around the party with the low rumble of voices in the background. Her feet carried her to Darnell sitting in the corner playing his guitar.

He smiled at her, saw her tears, and stopped his strumming. "Are you sad about Harriet?"

"Yes, but that's not why I'm crying."

He made room for her on the bench and patted the space he created. She sat with the realization that this was the one place she had wanted to sit all evening.

"Why the tears then?"

"I just found out my job is safe."

"Those don't look like tears of joy."

"I know. I don't know why I'm crying. My emotions are confusing. I wish I could control these damn tears…so embarrassing."

Darnell smiled. "I'm glad your job is safe. Tonight's a good time to cry. Everyone's crying."

Rachel sniffed and nodded her head. "I always thought of Ms. Leggett as rigid and mean, but now I see her as human and broken."

Darnell nodded. "Yeah, I see her insecurities when I'm on dialysis. I think that's why she hides in her office."

Rachel looked sideways at him, "So what else do you

observe from your dialysis chair?"

"I see courageous people living fragile and tenuous lives. I see people joking and laughing and taking care of each other." He said very quietly under his breath, "I see you."

Rachel couldn't make out the words he muttered under his breath but responded to his earlier sentences. "There's a lot of love in a dialysis unit."

They sat quietly for a few minutes before Rachel asked him, "Why are you hiding in this dark corner? Your guitar playing is beautiful."

"I didn't want to scare anyone with my monster face."

"You wouldn't scare a flea with your beautiful eyes. Did you get a chance to eat? Can I bring you some food?"

Darnell shook his head. "I prefer having you sitting next to me."

Rachel flushed. "I heard your mama talking to Howard about plans to pawn your motorcycle to raise bail for Will. Are those her plans, or yours?"

"She has been running her mouth about that plan since they locked Will up. Mama hates having him in jail. Personally, I think he is safer in there than out on the loose." He took a deep breath. "I'll consider Mama's plan when winter comes. I think Harold's pawn shop would be a nice, warm, dry place to store Rusty. I'm not willing to pawn her until November. October is the best time of year to ride."

"In the nursing universe we call them murder cycles. I bet your mama has other ulterior motives for pawning your motorcycle. She can keep both her sons safe with your motorcycle in the pawn shop."

Darnell nodded. "Mama hates Rusty, for that reason."

The line to say goodbye to Harriet became shorter, the party was thinning out, and the backyard grew quiet. Rachel saw Elizabeth and Martha take their places at the back of the line.

"I better go since Eli is my ride home. Do you want to get into the line with me to say goodbye to Harriet?"

He shook his head, "Nah, I told Harriet that I'd play until the end. When it's my turn, I'll tell her it's not too late to change her mind."

Rachel smiled, "Good luck with that."

Darnell touched her cheek as she got up to leave.

She felt his touch travel to her groin.

Darnell resumed his guitar playing and Rachel joined the line with Elizabeth. She watched the people in front of her saying goodbye. Harriet had something special to say to each person. Some goodbyes were tearful; others filled with laughter and hugs. She hugged each person from her wheelchair. Large people had a difficult time stooping low enough for her to get her little bony arms around their necks. Children climbed onto her wheelchair to say goodbye. Rachel realized that Harriet was using this time to bless each person individually one last time.

It was Elizabeth's turn to say goodbye. Rachel strained to hear what she was saying but only caught a word here and there. She heard Elizabeth thank her and she heard Harriet say something about being strong and courageous and taking one day at a time…something about her daughters also. She wondered what that was about.

When it was Rachel's turn, she noticed two remaining pieces of chocolate in Harriet's box of Malley's chocolates. Rachel pointed to the almost empty box and said, "Looks like you're enjoying that box of chocolates."

Harriet gave a slight giggle. "Yes, they're to die for. Would you like one?"

Flummoxed, Rachel shook her head. "No thanks."

Harriet asked Rachel to lean close. She placed her bony hands on both sides of Rachel's face and looked into her eyes.

"You are an excellent nurse. Trust God and don't be afraid of anything or anyone."

Rachel's eyes filled with tears at Harriet's words. She gave Harriet a hug and whispered in a hoarse voice, "God knows I'm going to miss you."

Elizabeth slung her arm over Rachel's shoulder as they walked to the car. Rachel continued crying. She said, "This is the first time in my life I've said goodbye to someone knowing that it was the last time. I'll never see Harriet alive again."

Elizabeth nodded. "Yeah, most of the time, we don't know that the last time is the last time. The night my husband died was just an ordinary night. I expected to wake up the next morning and see his face peeping over the newspaper at the breakfast table… A close friend of mine died suddenly, but I didn't know when we said goodbye that I'd never see her again. She was so full of life and plans. Those are big last times, but then there are the little ordinary last times that pass by unnoticed. There was a last time I read a book to my daughters at bedtime, tied a shoe for a soccer game, and a last time one of them needed my help with homework. Couldn't tell you when they happened. Hundreds of last times pass by unawares."

When they arrived at the car, both felt chilled.

"I'll turn the heat on as soon as the engine warms up a bit. First times are easier to recognize. This is the first time I'm turning the car heater on this season."

Rachel asked Eli if they could stop by the pharmacy to pick up a pregnancy test.

Eli looked at her sideways. "You think you might be pregnant?"

"I hope not, pregnancy isn't in our…Rachel used her two hands to make quotation marks 'marriage blueprint.' The plan is to wait five years before starting a family."

"Marriage blueprint? Does Steve think that life is plannable?"

"That, and he thinks it should conform to his idea of perfection. Lately, I've been wondering if I can live up to his expectations. I'm a mere human."

Elizabeth shook her head. "I'm afraid your beau is in for a rude awakening one of these days."

They drove in silence until Rachel brought up the revelation of Ms. Leggett being written up for a slow code. She asked Elizabeth why she hadn't told her earlier.

"I kept hoping Martha would tell you herself."

"That was slick how you brought it up in the conversation. Thanks."

"The suspense was killing me."

Rachel looked intently at Elizabeth. "Were you thinking I wouldn't ask Ms. Leggett about the investigation?"

"Would you have?"

"I wanted to, every day I planned to, but I always managed to talk myself out of it. I guess I'm afraid of her. Harriet told me not to be afraid of anything or anyone. Easier said than done."

Elizabeth nodded. "I understand being afraid to bring something up. I have something important to discuss with my daughters. Every day I say to myself, 'Today is the day,' and I don't follow through."

Rachel waited silently, hoping Elizabeth would elaborate further. When she didn't, she asked quietly, "Would you like to discuss it with me?"

Elizabeth hesitated, and then blurted out, "I'm in late stage four kidney failure and have chosen not to do dialysis. Every day at work, I see a future I don't want. I plan to have a party like Harriet and die a natural death with lots of high-potassium foods and maybe too much insulin."

It had been a night for tears and Rachel started crying again and shook her head. "No, no. I need you. Don't go. You need to stay. I need you to stay around. I understand why you were afraid to tell your daughters. They need you more than I do."

Elizabeth replied in a motherly tone, "I don't know when my kidneys will fail to the point of needing dialysis. I may have a few years, maybe longer. Only God knows. Life was simpler before the miracles of modern medicine. Everyone knew they would die sometime and died a natural death."

Rachel hesitated before saying through her tears, "I've noticed that you haven't been your usual lively self lately."

"The energy is gone. Some days suck everything out of me."

Elizabeth waited in the car as Rachel walked into the twenty-four-hour fluorescent pharmacy. Rachel continued crying, one grief on top of another. She would have preferred to purchase a pregnancy test under the cover of darkness, especially with her blotchy, swollen face, but then she suspected the cashiers were accustomed to seeing tearful women purchasing pregnancy tests.

Pregnancy tests lined the shelf: AccuClear, Clear Blue Digital Pregnancy Test with Smart Countdown, First Response Early Result Pregnancy Test and more. So many options. She ended up picking the cheapest and smallest test that could be hidden in her purse. She planned to hide this entire enterprise from Steve, at least until she knew the results.

- Chapter 25 -

Elizabeth loved Sunday mornings. She loafed in her pajamas as she read the *Sunday Plain Dealer*, drank coffee, and munched a scone or two. She opened the newspaper to the 'Health Beat' first, to read what her daughter Becky had written. This week's topic was black-market organ transplants. When Elizabeth saw the title, she poured herself a second cup of coffee and put her reading glasses on.

Becky's article started with the explanation that a kidney transplant is the gold standard treatment for a person with end-stage kidney disease (ESKD). With a functioning kidney, a person can live a normal life without suffering the complications and inconveniences of dialysis. The problem is, there aren't enough kidneys for everyone who needs one.

There are different options for obtaining a kidney. The best option is a living-related transplant from a close relative who matches. Living-related transplants last the longest. Many people though, don't have relatives willing or able to donate a kidney. The second-best transplant option is a living non-related transplant. These transplants occur when a person has a close friend or relative who wants to donate their kidney. Occasionally, it can be a good match, but other times the donor's blood doesn't match the recipient's blood. Clever schemes have been devised to get around that problem. Transplant centers can arrange for a paired exchange, otherwise known as a kidney swap. In these cases, the willing donor can give their kidney to someone who is a better match, and the person they wanted to give their kidney to receives a kidney from someone else who is also a better match. Sometimes paired exchanges get very elaborate, with up to six or eight people involved in a kidney donation chain.

The third and most common option is a deceased donor transplant. These kidneys are procured from someone who was healthy but died suddenly, usually from an accident of some kind. Patients on kidney transplant waiting lists are waiting for these kidneys. There are over 120,000 patients on the transplant waiting list in the US. The average wait time is four years, but for many patients the wait can stretch much longer.

After reviewing the basics of kidney transplantation, Becky's article addressed the black-market trade in kidneys. She wrote that it is illegal to sell an organ anywhere in the world, except for Iran. However, the lack of enforcement in many countries, makes it easy to offer financial incentives to poor people to part with their kidneys. Black market hot spots for kidneys change over time depending upon the ever-changing politics and power structures in countries.

The problem of transplant tourism waned after the 'Declaration of Istanbul Against Global Organ Exploitation' was signed in 2008 by over 100 nephrology groups and countries. However, the problem mushroomed again due to an increased international demand for organs and greed. In 2016, Pope Francis listed organ trafficking as one of the 'new forms of slavery' and true crimes against humanity.

The article stated that there are over 10,000 black market transplants each year worldwide: approximately one illegal transplant per hour. The Istanbul conference had established a "Custodian Group": a network of physicians around the world that report to each other whenever there is a suspected case of organ trafficking. In the article, Becky quoted Cleveland nephrologist Dr. Max Burnouf, who is a member of the Custodian Group.

When Elizabeth saw his name in the article, she gasped. "I

didn't know he was active in fighting organ trafficking. I wonder if he could have intervened with Marguerite?"

Dr Burnouf described a recent dialysis patient who had gone to Mexico for a black-market transplant. When the patient's body rejected the kidney and it had to be removed, they discovered that this older woman had been transplanted with a child's kidney. The surgeons estimated that the child was approximately ten years old.

Dr Burnouf suspected the kidney originated with the Mexican drug cartels, who had recently started dabbling in organ trafficking. The steady wave of refugees pouring out of Central America, hoping to escape violence in their home countries, had become what he called a "migrant holocaust." Mexican cartels kidnap the most helpless and vulnerable of those seeking asylum – mere children – and take them to rented homes with medical equipment and remove their organs. Dr. Burnouf said that he could not be sure, but he suspected a helpless refugee child was the source of his patient's kidney. Dr. Burnouf wondered if other organs were removed and if the child was still alive.

Elizabeth's eyes teared when she read this. "How could anyone do this to a child?" She pictured Max sitting at his desk with his head in his hands. Her heart ached. She grabbed her cell phone to call him but remembered that she was avoiding him, and they weren't talking. She missed him.

Since Max Burnouf was out of the question, she called Becky, who didn't pick up. After leaving a message, she called Rachel. "Rachel, do you get the Plain Dealer?"

"No, why?"

"My daughter Becky wrote an article in the 'Health Beat' about black market kidney transplants. In the article she quoted Max, who discussed a patient who obtained one in Mexico. I bet it was Marguerite. I'll bring the article for you to read tomorrow. I wish I could have stopped Marguerite from doing it… So, what did the pregnancy test show?"

"I was afraid to check it today. I'm scheduled to open the unit tomorrow, so I'll be up before 4:00 am. I'll do the test while Steve sleeps."

"Okay, see you tomorrow."

Elizabeth lounged around for a few more hours as she read the rest of the paper. She started her laundry and did some housecleaning. Sunday afternoons used to be more exciting when Ebony was alive. Elizabeth and Ebony would go for long walks at a nearby park. Ebony helped her to ignore the mountains of dirty laundry and dust bunnies dancing under the furniture.

At 2:00 pm, as she was putting the final load of laundry away, her two daughters showed up at her front door. Elizabeth hugged them with glee at the surprise visit, but they responded stiffly to her embrace. Elizabeth told Becky that she left a voicemail for her after reading her article and was so happy she was here so they could discuss it.

Her daughters walked past her with heads lowered and sat on the living room couch next to each other, holding hands. It looked like they had been crying.

Lauren said in a low voice, "We need to talk to you, Mom."

Elizabeth sat in the chair across from the sofa, leaned forward and asked, "What happened? Are you both okay? Did something happen to one of your boyfriends?"

Becky shook her head and said in a testy voice, "No Mom, *you* need to tell *us* what's going on." Becky told her that in the process of interviewing Dr. Burnouf, he told her about Elizabeth's plans to forgo dialysis and die.

Elizabeth raised her voice. "Max told you that? That's illegal. A HIPAA violation."

"Mom," they both howled in unison and then started talking at once. "Were you ever going to tell us? Shouldn't we be a part of your decision? We're your family. Your choices and decisions affect us. You never even told us your kidneys were going bad."

Elizabeth felt ambushed; her cheeks grew hot as she leaned back on her chair. "I planned to discuss this with you; I was just waiting for the right opportunity. I didn't know how to start the conversation. I wanted to spare you the pain you experienced when Dad died."

Becky snapped, "Mom, this pain is worse. Your death would be pre-meditated. Dad would never have chosen to leave us."

Lauren took a more measured and reasoned approach. "If you can't discuss this with us, who can you discuss it with?"

Elizabeth sighed, "I knew you both looked to me to be strong and in control after Dad died. I really wanted to discuss it with you, really, but I didn't know how."

Lauren replied in a soft voice, "You were the best mom ever, and we appreciate everything you did for us when we were little, but now we're adults, not your little girls anymore. We don't need you to be strong. We don't need your protection anymore. Tell us everything."

Elizabeth nodded and spoke in fits and starts. She felt shame admitting to her daughters that her body was failing.

She told them that diabetes had caused damage all over her body.

She had nerve damage and poor circulation in her legs and feet. Her feet were numb and sometimes very painful. She worried about an amputation or two in her future. She had watched so many patients lose their legs inch by inch.

Her eyesight was deteriorating, and she was afraid of going blind and not being able to drive herself anymore.

She described her fatigue, how the days were getting harder, and finally, how her kidneys were failing.

Then she told them about dialysis patients that she had known over the years. She wanted to spare her daughters the pain of watching her slow decline. "I don't want you two pushing me in a wheelchair from one doctor's appointment to another. I don't want your last memories of me to be of wiping my butt or reminding me of your names."

Lauren and Becky listened intently as their mom laid it all out.

Lauren said, "Mom, we didn't know. We're so sorry you are going through this."

Elizabeth sighed and relaxed against the chair back. "Thank God you understand. I'm relieved to finally get it off my chest."

Lauren replied calmly as both shook their heads. "We understand how you feel, but we don't accept your choice."

Becky teared up. "Mom, Joe and I are getting married. Who will be the mother of the bride? Who will be a grandma to our kids?"

Elizabeth smiled. "You two are getting married? I liked Joe the moment I met him. Such a wonderful man. Have you set a date? So much fun to plan a wedding."

"Our wedding is not on the table today. Dr. Burnouf told me that it's time for you to get a dialysis access because it's impossible to predict when your kidneys will stop working completely. He wants you to be prepared. He thinks you might be depressed."

Elizabeth rolled her eyes. "He thinks everyone's depressed… he has a good friend who is a psychiatrist. I think they may have a little kickback scheme going between the two of them."

Lauren groaned. "Mom, that's crazy talk. I bet a lot of kidney patients struggle with depression. It's nothing to be ashamed of."

Becky interjected. "We're not leaving today until you agree to get a dialysis access."

Elizabeth sighed and rubbed her eyes. She stared at the floor as the clock on the mantle chimed. She stood and opened a window. "It's getting warm in here, don't you think?" She sat again and rubbed her palms up and down her thighs before taking a deep breath. "There is no rush. There's plenty of time to discuss this further with you. There are lots of options for treating kidney disease, and 'no dialysis' is a valid option."

Becky interjected, "Not according to Dr. Burnouf. He told me that you are probably looking at dialysis or death within the year, and sometimes it can take up to six months for a dialysis fistula to mature."

Elizabeth looked at Becky and squinted her eyes. "How much time did you spend talking with Dr. Burnouf about me?"

Becky tilted her head. "Well, he spent fifteen minutes discussing his patient with the black-market kidney, and forty-five minutes discussing you. He considers us family; you worked together for so many years. I think he always hoped that one of us would marry one of his sons." Becky shot a knowing glance at Lauren.

Lauren said, "Mom, the tides have changed. It's our turn to take care of you."

Becky handed her mother an appointment slip. "Dr Burnouf's secretary made you an appointment with the best vascular surgeon in Cleveland. It's two weeks from now on one of your days off. We both took the day off work to attend the appointment with you."

"You're trying to control my life."

Lauren smiled. "We used to say that to you when you wouldn't allow us to get tattoos, or go to frat parties in high school, or when you forbade us to hang around with Jonathan and his druggie friends."

Becky stood and marched around her mother's chair, waving her hands in the air. "You were *so* controlling… making us do our homework…eat our vegetables…and take ballet lessons."

Lauren administered the coup de grace: "Mom, you always tell us that you love us and will do anything for us. If you really mean it, take a chance at life and try dialysis. Do it for us."

Becky said, "Dr. Burnouf told me that you have options. You can do peritoneal dialysis on your own at home. If you choose home hemodialysis, we can be your partners, and you wouldn't even have to go to a dialysis unit. Joe and I could move in with you and help you."

"No one is moving in with me." Elizabeth sighed. "I love you both more than my own life. I shouldn't have to *do* dialysis to prove my love for you, but I will. I do however reserve the right to stop dialysis if I become too sick or start to lose who I am."

Becky sat across from her mother and leaned forward. "Mom, you wouldn't have to do dialysis forever. Dr. Burnouf told me that if you lose thirty pounds, one of us can give you a kidney. That's how much we love you."

Elizabeth started crying. Becky and Lauren walked to their mother's chair, sat on each armrest and put their arms around her.

When Elizabeth stopped crying, she stood and said, "I'd planned to take you both to that new wine bistro around the corner to discuss my no-dialysis decision, but I kept putting it off. Are you both free to come with me this afternoon? We need to plan a wedding."

Becky replied, "We cleared our schedules for the afternoon. We know how stubborn you are and expected this discussion to take a lot longer. You were easier than we thought."

As they headed out the door, with Elizabeth's two daughters leading the way, Elizabeth heard Lauren whisper to her sister, "Wait until she finds out what else we have up our sleeves."

She grabbed both daughters by the backs of their hoodies, shoved them slightly and said, "You two are in big trouble. We'll discuss your punishment at the wine bistro."

The two sisters gave each other a high five.

- Chapter 26 -

Rachel climbed out of bed at 3:30 am Monday morning. She glanced at the calendar on her phone and saw that today marked the fall equinox. This is the day the earth shifts on its axis to darker, colder, and more grueling days. She shivered in the chilly morning air and noticed that Rosh Hashanah was a week away. Steve's family was coming to their home for the holiday dinner for the first time ever. In the past, Steve's mother Miriam always hosted the holidays, but she was undergoing last-ditch chemotherapy for recurrent breast cancer. She remembered days of laughter in Miriam's kitchen, learning to cook with Steve's sister Maxine. She didn't want to think of Miriam being gone.

She fished the pregnancy test out of her purse and read the directions. Her hands shook as she attempted to pee on the wand. The wand slipped out of her hands and clattered against the porcelain toilet. *Shit! I hope that didn't wake Steve.* Two wands came with the test kit, and she wondered if dropping the first test was a common occurrence. She fished the wand out of the toilet, wrapped it in toilet paper, and discarded it before attempting the second test. This time she gripped it tightly as she obtained the urine sample.

She showered as the test analyzed her future. As she lathered her hair, she repeated this mantra: *God, please let it be negative. Let it be negative. Let it be negative. Let it be negative...* When she finished her shower, she looked at the wand on the counter and saw a pink plus sign indicating pregnancy. Her stomach dropped. She closed her eyes as a wave of nausea hit her. *Oy vey iz mir.* She sat on the toilet with her head in her hands until the wave of nausea passed. She hoped it was a false positive. She couldn't remember missing any birth control pills and hoped the problem was the cheap pregnancy test. She planned to pick up a better test on the way home from work today.

At 4:30 am, she arrived at the dialysis unit; the lights glowed through the windows as she parked in the dark. Inside the unit, machines hummed and buzzed as the technicians rushed around preparing the unit for the first shift of patients arriving at 5:30 am. The technicians always arrived before the nurses because it was their responsibility to prepare the dialysate, the salt and electrolyte solution needed to clean patients' blood. Strict protocols dictate the steps necessary to ensure the safety of the dialysate. During a dialysis treatment, a patient's blood is exposed to approximately one hundred liters of dialysate. A few stray bacteria, too many electrolytes, chlorine, heavy metals, or other contaminates in the water can kill a patient or several patients simultaneously in the same unit.

Rachel walked into the bustling unit and shouted good morning to everyone as the phone rang. It was one of Harriet's daughters reporting that her mom had passed quietly and comfortably early Sunday morning.

Rachel sat and took a deep breath. "Her memory will always be a blessing for everyone who knew her." Rachel offered condolences and said she would let everyone in the unit know.

Harriet's daughter replied, "We miss her already. We're still cleaning up the yard after her going away party. One minute, we're crying, another minute laughing, remembering, and reliving her final hours. She was so full of life and love until the end."

Rachel hung up and thought of Harriet before reviewing the patient schedule for the day. She was stunned to discover that the new patient assigned to Harriet's chair was Marguerite, of all people. She reviewed Marguerite's chart notes from the hospital, read about her transplant rejection, and the attempts to salvage the transplanted kidney. She also read about her resuscitation and ICU stay. Rachel updated Marguerite's dialysis electronic chart with the new dialysis orders and the stats from her last dialysis in the hospital. She wondered what drama Marguerite would bring to the unit. She had been so difficult and disruptive previously.

Tamika was assigned to Marguerite's pod this month. Rachel remembered the time Marguerite humiliated Tamika when she wouldn't allow her to insert her needles because of her 'fat butt.' In the months since Ethel's death, Rachel's relationship with Tamika had settled into a cold truce. They spoke with each other politely when necessary for patient care, and Tamika had stopped badmouthing Rachel in front of patients. The situation was tolerable but still uncomfortable. Today Rachel saw an opportunity to improve their relation-ship. She approached Tamika with the schedule, pointed to Marguerite's name in Harriet's old chair and shook her head. They made eye contact for the first time in months, perhaps the first time ever.

Rachel said, "I'm sorry you're stuck with her today. Her Mexican kidney nearly did her in. Harriet wanted me to make sure the corner group welcomed the new person in her chair."

Tamika's lips pursed as she shook her head. "Good luck with that."

"I'll meet her at the door and do the initial assessment. Let me know if you have any problems. I've got your back. She's not allowed to abuse you."

Fifteen minutes later, Marguerite hobbled in using a walker with her husband carrying her belongings. In the past she had either driven herself or her husband had dropped her off at the entrance and sped away.

Marguerite had always been thin, but now she had become skeletal; a frail, pale caricature of her previously bitchy, impe-rial self. Her hair was frizzy, and she had a two-inch line of gray roots dividing her red bushy hair. Rachel had a fleeting impression of an aged Bozo the clown without his makeup and big smile. Marguerite's shirt tented her frame, and the skin on her arms hung loosely; the loose diamond ring on her finger threatened to slip off. Marguerite held her sweatpants with one hand to keep them from sliding off her bottom. Rachel touched her arm and lied, "Welcome back Marguerite. It's nice to see you again." She weighed Marguerite and noted that she had lost twenty pounds since her last dialysis session in the unit before her Mexican adventure. As she walked Marguerite to Harriet's old chair, Marguerite stopped shuffling and asked what happened to Harriet.

"She withdrew from dialysis and died yesterday."

Marguerite shook her head. "She kept everyone in the unit going."

That Marguerite had even been aware of Harriet's existence startled Rachel. Everyone in the unit knew Marguerite, but Marguerite had ignored everyone. Tamika was busy setting up the machine and said hi to Marguerite but kept her back towards her.

Rachel examined Marguerite and found that though she had lost weight, she still had more water weight to lose. Her blood pressure was elevated, there were crackles in her lungs, and her legs and feet were swollen. Rachel knew Marguerite's true dry weight was much less than the weight obtained on the scale a few minutes earlier. Her fistula still worked. Marguerite denied being short of breath, denied chest pain, and said she could sleep comfortably. Rachel advised Tamika to set the dialysis machine to remove two kg. of fluid, but to check her blood pressure every fifteen minutes and watch her carefully, because this was her first session back in the unit and they would need to gradually discover her new dry weight.

Rachel started rounding on the other patients but watched Marguerite out of the corner of her eye, hoping that she would be kind to Tamika.

A few hours later, Elizabeth moseyed in. She looked better than she had for weeks. She told Rachel that her daughters had strong-armed her into agreeing to get an access for dialysis.

Rachel did a fist pump. "Yessss! I knew I liked your daughters the first time I met them."

"They gave me too many reasons to circle the sun a few more times. Becky is getting married. Now I'll have to deal with my fear of needles and watching my blood circulating in tubes outside my body."

"You've got to be kidding. You have diabetes, have been a nurse for over forty years, working in dialysis for at least twenty of those years, and you're afraid of needles and blood?"

Elizabeth grinned sheepishly. "I confess. I am not afraid of all needles; just large ones pointed in my direction. Don't tell anybody, I'll be the laughingstock of the unit. Here is the article on organ trafficking that I told you about."

Rachel took the newspaper article, folded it, and stuffed it in her pocket. She whispered to Elizabeth that Marguerite was in Harriet's old chair, nodding her head in Marguerite's direction. "She is a shadow of her former self. We are trying to take some extra fluid off. I'll be anxious to hear your opinion after you examine her."

Elizabeth asked Rachel about the pregnancy test.

"It was positive, but I'm hoping it's wrong. I'll pick up another test kit at the pharmacy on the way home from work today."

"False negative pregnancy tests happen, but rarely false positives. I'm sensing this isn't a welcome development?"

She shook her head. "I'm not expecting a congratulatory 'Mazel Tov' from Steve. He'll blame me even though I took birth control pills religiously. I don't think I missed a single pill."

"I'll say 'Mazel Tov' then. You'll be a great mom. A child will take you places in your life and heart that you can't even imagine. I'm volunteering to be a surrogate grandmother to your child."

"I'll take you up on that offer. My mother doesn't want grandchildren. When Steve and I announced our engagement, the first words out of my mom's mouth were, 'Don't make me a grandmother.' Not that any children of mine would lose out. She's a master at judgment and criticism, not so much love and comfort. Sometimes it takes me a week to recover from a visit with her."

Elizabeth tilted her head. "What do you think made your mom so mean?"

"Her parents were Holocaust survivors. I know her childhood was grim. I can look at her circumstances and understand how they made her who she is, but another part of me has a hard time forgiving her for being so mean to me. I'm not as awful as she says I am. My father's early death didn't help. I became an expense and burden to her."

Elizabeth asked, "What about Steve's parents? Will they be looking forward to grandparenting?"

"Steve's mom is fighting a losing battle with a recurrence of breast cancer. I don't expect her to be around much longer. His dad is aloof."

Rachel noticed Tamika leaving her pod and heading to the tech area. "Excuse me, Eli. I want to make sure things are going well with Marguerite and Tamika."

When she reached Tamika, she asked, "Any updates on our 'new' patient?"

Tamika smiled. "Marguerite keeps apologizing for her cruelty to me. I feel like I'm in a sci-fi movie where aliens inhabit human bodies. I want to ask her, 'Who are you? And what have you done with Marguerite?'"

Rachel laughed. "Seeing Marguerite sitting in Harriet's chair turns my world upside down too." She pulled Elizabeth's article from her pocket. "Eli brought in this article about organ trafficking. She thinks it may be about Marguerite. I'll read it during my break and leave it on the bulletin board for whoever else wants to read it. Something terrible must have happened with the transplant."

Tamika replied, "Yeah, I'd say something happened. I heard her tell Mattie that not only was it a bad decision to get the transplant, but an evil one, and she wished she had never done it."

During her lunch break, Rachel read the *Plain Dealer* article on organ trafficking and felt incredibly sad for Marguerite and the child donor. As she pinned the article on the bulletin board, she noticed that Ms. Leggett (Martha as she now thought of her) had posted the letter from Peter Swanson, the Regional Technical Director, commending Rachel for identifying the problem with machine number twenty-three. She felt exposed, not wanting the attention, but also felt a slight twinge of pride. She wondered if Martha was trying to make amends for letting her sweat for weeks about losing her job.

Shortly after that, Darnell arrived for his shift. Rachel always tried to act detached and professional when caring for him but found herself sneaking glances at him at different times, sometimes discovering that he was looking at her already. Usually, their eyes met for the briefest of seconds, but today he winked at her.

Darnell, J.R., and Mr. Freeman had become co-conspirators in plotting activities each dialysis session to get Rachel's attention; often calling her over with inane questions and problems. While she rounded on every patient, these three called her over two to three extra times during a shift for their entertainment and enjoyment. Their objective was to get her to laugh and to keep her at their chairs longer than the usual time. Sometimes she indulged them; other days she ignored them to finish her work.

Today, Darnell posed the question, "Inquiring minds want to know. What happened to Marguerite in Mexico?

J.R. said, "It looks like she's aged twenty years. We were expecting her to be dancing around the unit with maracas. Tell us the story, the unabridged version."

Mr. Freeman said, "She looks like a concentration camp survivor."

"You guys have tried this before and should know by now that I can't talk to you about other patients. I can't talk to Mr. Freeman about J.R.; I can't even speak to Darnell's mama about him. Why don't you ask her yourself? She may want to tell you the story."

The three conspirators didn't like her suggestion; it was hard for them to admit it, but they were afraid of Marguerite's sharp tongue.

When Rachel walked away, the three men beckoned Tamika to their chairs. Tamika obliged and stood there for a good five minutes talking with them.

When she walked away from them, Rachel wandered over to her nonchalantly and said, "I hope you didn't give them any information about Marguerite. You know that would be a HIPAA violation."

"I know more than you give me credit for. I didn't say a word about Marguerite. I spent the whole time talking about you." She grinned. "I told them about the letter commending you on the bulletin board. I told them that initially I thought you were just being superstitious about machine number twenty-three."

"What???"

"I told them that I admired your persistence."

Rachel's cheeks got hot. "I can only wish that were a HIPAA violation, then you'd be in deep trouble."

- Chapter 27 -

Rachel decided not to get a repeat pregnancy test after Eli told her that false positive pregnancy tests are rare. She figured Steve would probably insist on repeating it with the best test on the market anyway. On the drive home she tried to figure out the best way to let Steve know she was pregnant. She had no idea how far along she was. *How do I tell him? How long can I wait until he starts seeing my belly getting larger? I need to tell him soon, like tonight.*

She hoped he would relish the idea of becoming a father. Perhaps parenthood would change the dynamics of their relationship. Then her thoughts vacillated from hopes about Steve to fears about her competence as a mother. She couldn't keep houseplants alive, and she didn't learn any mothering skills from her own mother.

Her thoughts drifted to Steve's mother. After her conversation with Elizabeth, she realized that she had been suppressing her awareness of Steve's mother's battle with cancer. She wondered if that was what was bothering Steve, wondered if he was grieving over his mother's impending death and unaware of it.

She walked into the house to find Steve stretched out on the couch watching baseball. Rachel greeted him, "Hi Honey. Who's winning?"

"It's the sixth inning and the score is nothing–nothing."

"A good reminder of why I hate baseball. I went to a Cleveland opener with my best friend and her mother when I was fourteen. That game lasted sixteen innings. After that, I lost any desire to watch another baseball game again in my life."

"You think baseball is boring. Your high school soccer games were deadly; watching girls kick a soccer ball back and forth, back and forth, back and forth, for two hours with nothing happening."

She felt the dig but changed the subject, "So how was your day?"

"I started doing research on your patient, Daniel."

"His name's Darnell."

"Darnell, Daniel…What's the difference? I have discovered that it may be more difficult to win his case than I initially thought."

"That's what your colleagues said at the cocktail party. Something about the doctrine of 'qualified immunity.' Can you find another angle? Maybe not sue the individual cops but the police department or the city? Perhaps they didn't train the cops as well as they should have?"

"I'll keep working on an angle. Those cops did a number on him. What's for dinner?"

Rachel felt so, so, so tired. "I need to take a nap. Wake me up when the game is over. Maybe we can eat out tonight."

Rachel removed her shoes and scrubs and collapsed on top of the comforter with just her underwear on. She woke to the sound of thunder and Steve sitting on the edge of the bed in his underwear. She smiled and stretched. Lightning lit up the room with thunder exploding seconds later. Rain poured in sheets down the windowpanes.

Rachel sat up and continued to stretch a little more. "I don't suppose these are ideal weather conditions for going out to eat."

Steve touched her lips and cheek gently, then ran his fingers from her chin, down her midline, and rested his hand on her lower abdomen. "These are perfect conditions for what I'm hungry for now."

Warmth and heaviness filled Rachel's lower body. He

took her face into both his hands and kissed her hungrily, his tongue probing her mouth. Full of desire, and wet already, she slipped off her bra and underwear and helped Steve remove his underwear. She massaged his genitals before straddling him. Their lovemaking started slowly and gently, gradually increasing in rhythm and intensity until they both orgasmed simultaneously. Steve came with a shudder and a loud exclamation, Rachel with a low moan. They collapsed breathless on the bed still embracing.

They cuddled as the storm subsided.

Rachel turned towards him. "This may be the last thunderstorm of the season. Today is the Fall Equinox."

Steve, half dozing, his lips against her shoulder, just mumbled, "Mhmmm."

Eventually, Rachel sat up. "I'm hungry. Let's go to the Mediterranean restaurant around the corner."

The night air was cool and dark. Trees spit large raindrops when the wind blew. They held hands as they huddled under their umbrella and walked to the restaurant. Rachel hoped that Steve, mellowed by sex, would be receptive to discussing her pregnancy. *Perfect timing.*

The waiter led them to a corner table with a candle flickering. The restaurant was quiet with a few patrons finishing their meals. As they scanned the menu, Steve asked Rachel if he should order the usual glass of Merlot for her. She continued reading the menu. "No thanks."

"Well, what can I order you? Would you like a martini, a marguerita, a daiquiri, a mojito?"

"None of the above. I think I may be pregnant." *There, I said it.*

He jerked his head and looked at her. "What?"

"Well, remember how I couldn't fit into the cocktail dress? Then I started thinking how lately my breasts have been tender and I've been so tired. Those are pregnancy symptoms. So,

I took a pregnancy test this morning, and it came out positive."

"Could it be a mistake?"

"False positive pregnancy tests are rare."

"Make an appointment for an abortion."

She tilted her head and shook it slightly. "An abortion?" Rachel's body tensed.

He raised his voice enough so that the remaining restaurant patrons could hear, "Now is not the right time to have a family. Don't sabotage our five-year plan. Get an abortion. We can have children when we're ready."

Rachel leaned forward and hissed, "I took my birth control pills religiously. If you were so worried about having children, you should have used condoms."

Steve whispered harshly to keep her voice down, even though it was his deep voice that echoed in the restaurant. He said through gritted teeth, "You need to get an abortion." The few remaining restaurant patrons stopped eating their desserts and gaped at the drama unfolding before them.

Rachel sat silently, squeezing her lower lip and folding it between her thumb and forefinger. She watched him drinking his martini. *How can he be so callous and mean? He's putting abortion in the same category as discarding a piece of furniture or selling a stock option. He thinks he can order me around, like I have no say in the matter.* She was pro-choice in politics, knowing some of the desperate circumstances that women find themselves in, but never considered abortion a reasonable choice for herself. She sat silently for a long time, staring at the menu.

Eventually Steve demanded, "So, are you going to make the appointment or not?"

Overwhelmed with sadness, she sighed. "I'll call my GYN tomorrow."

"Good. That's my girl. So, what are you going to order for dinner?"

Rachel had lost her appetite. "I think I'll just order a bowl of soup."

Rachel sulked for the rest of the meal. The soup tasted salty, and the vegetables mushy. She made no attempt at further conversation. Steve downed two martinis as he finished his meal. Rachel hated the sound of his chewing and slurping. They walked home in silence, no longer holding hands, and abandoning the umbrella at the restaurant.

- Chapter 28 -

The first OB-GYN appointment Rachel could get with Dr. Mary O'Keefe was the last appointment of the day on the Eve of Rosh Hashanah. Rachel spent the entire day preparing a feast with beef brisket, fruit compote, matzah ball soup, green bean casserole, and noodle kugel. She wanted it to be special for Miriam, a thank-you for everything she had taught her. Rachel set the dining room table with fine linens, china, silverware, and candles, taking pains to make everything beautiful for Steve's family. The dinner preparations took longer than expected. She put the dinner into the oven on warm before rushing to her OB-GYN appointment with a jittery stomach. She had intended to stop at the bakery on her way to the appointment but figured that she could stop on the way home.

Dr. O'Keefe walked into the exam room with a piece of paper in her hand. "Hello Rachel, congratulations! You're pregnant."

Rachel shook her head slightly. "I don't think I missed a single pill."

Dr. O'Keefe sat down at the desk. "I'm sensing this pregnancy is unplanned."

"I keep trying to figure out how it happened?"

"No birth control method is one hundred percent fail-safe."

"I remember a time a few months back when I had a GI bug and couldn't keep my food down for two days. I took the pill those days, but perhaps it came back up with the rest of my stomach contents. Could I have become pregnant then?"

"I can't say for sure, but that's a good possibility." Dr.

O'Keefe probed, "Since this pregnancy wasn't planned, are you considering abortion?"

Rachel looked at the floor. "My fiancé wants me to get one. I don't know."

"Hmmm. That's a problem. Don't get one to please your partner. Often, relationships disintegrate when there is discord, with one person wanting an abortion and the other not wanting it. Let's find out how far along you are. That will give us an idea of your options."

Dr. O'Keefe reviewed Rachel's medical history and examined her. She estimated her to be twelve weeks along. She performed an ultrasound to confirm the dates and ensure the fetus was developing properly. Rachel watched the ultrasound, unable to interpret the indistinct gray moving shadows. Her doctor pointed to the fetal heart, head, and limbs. It was mysterious and awesome. Dr. O'Keefe handed her a picture of the ultrasound to take home. She estimated her due date to be mid-April.

Dr. O'Keefe again broached the subject of abortion. "I am afraid that you are too far along in your pregnancy for the abortion pill to be effective. Your fiancé wants an abortion, but you are undecided. I know a good counselor to help you decide. She also does joint counseling if your fiancé is interested."

Rachel mutely nodded her head.

"What you need to know is that you don't have much time to make this decision, just a few weeks. Ohio law requires two visits for an abortion, and they require another ultrasound."

When Rachel found her voice, she told Dr. O'Keefe she had a lot to think about. Dr. O'Keefe advised her to make a follow-up appointment in a month. If she had an abortion, she would still want to see her and make sure she was healing well; if she kept the pregnancy, she would make sure things were progressing as they should. Dr. O'Keefe gave Rachel a prescription for prenatal vitamins and instructed her to avoid alcohol, eat well, get plenty of rest, and moderate exercise… the usual.

Rachel walked out of the doctor's office filled with uncertainty. It was late September, and the tips of the leaves on the maple trees were dipped in blood. *It's not just trees changing. I'll never be the same.*

Rachel stopped at the bakery on the way home to pick up challah and honey cake for the evening's celebration. She discovered a long line and the counter lady working in slow motion. She wore heavy black eyeliner and had a thick accent from some Eastern European country. She struggled to understand customer orders and figure out the change. A five-minute errand stretched into a forty-minute agony.

When she finally arrived home, she saw Steve's parents' car parked in front of the house. *Shit, I'm late.* She drove to the little turnaround in the back of the house and rushed through the rear kitchen door. She unloaded the bakery bags, the ultrasound picture, and the prenatal vitamin prescription on the kitchen countertop before scrambling with the final dinner touches, placing the challah on the bread platter, covering it with the challah cover, and setting it on the dining room table. She quickly placed cut apples and honey at each place setting (A Rosh Hashanah tradition wishing for a sweet new year) before turning on the stove to reheat the broth for the matzah ball soup. Steve, his parents, and younger sister Maxine sat in the living room talking quietly.

Rachel rushed in to welcome her guests and wish them all L'Shana Tovah. "I'm sorry I'm late, the lady from Kazakhstan or wherever manned the counter at the bakery and took forever."

Steve's sister Maxine commiserated with her, "I was in her line yesterday afternoon." Steve's father and sister stood up to give Rachel a hug. Rachel hugged Steve's mother in the chair so she wouldn't have to stand.

As she hugged her, she said, "I'm so glad you could make it today. How are you feeling?"

"As good as can be expected. Thank you for making this celebration for all of us. We are drooling over the aromas wafting in from the kitchen."

"All your recipes…if it weren't for you teaching me how to cook, I'd be boiling hot dogs for Rosh Hashanah. Everything's ready." She helped Miriam get out of her chair and led her carefully into the dining room. The family stood around the table as Rachel lit the candles, marking the transition from a profane time to a sacred time. The dining room emanated a quiet, holy, golden glow from the candles and the setting sun. Silverware and plates sparkled in the candlelight. Steve said the prayers over the bread and wine in Hebrew. The family dipped their apples in the honey and prayed together, "May it be Your Will to bless us with a good and sweet year." Rachel prayed silently for her future mother-in-law, "Please heal Miriam."

After everyone sat, Rachel said, "The matzah ball soup is hot."

Maxine assisted Rachel in the kitchen. Rachel dispensed the soup into the bowls as Maxine carried them to the table. When Maxine came for the last bowl of Matzah ball soup, she noticed the ultrasound picture lying on the counter and picked it up. "What is this?" Then her smile broadened. "Oh, I know." Before Rachel could stop her or explain, Maxine exclaimed, "Mazel Tov," and ran into the dining room waving the picture in her hand. "Mama and Papa, you are about to become grandparents!"

Rachel followed her reluctantly, carrying the last bowl of matzah ball soup for herself.

There was a mixed response to Maxine's happy announcement. Steve became even more stony-faced than when Rachel arrived late.

Miriam expressed concern. "I know you're planning on

getting married next May, but have you two discussed moving the wedding up?"

Rachel stared at the matzah ball floating in the chicken broth. "This pregnancy is unexpected. We were taking precautions. Sort of throws a wrench into everything, doesn't it?" She caught Miriam's eyes.

Miriam smiled. "Well, the good thing is that perhaps I'll still have the blessing of holding my first grandchild before I die."

Steve's father just grunted and slurped his matzah ball soup. He was a man of few words except when it came to sports. At that point, Steve announced that he had instructed Rachel to get an abortion because it wasn't the right time to start a family.

Everyone turned to look at him, their faces registering varying degrees of shock. The holy atmosphere from the candle lighting dissipated.

"Stevie darling, it's not just your decision," Miriam remonstrated. "A decision like this should be made jointly, but even so, Rachel should have the final say." She shrugged her shoulders. "Also, inconvenient as this pregnancy is, perhaps it is meant to be?" She turned to Rachel. "What are your thoughts on this?"

Rachel, still staring at her matzah ball, shook her head and mumbled, "I don't know."

Steve's father tried to lighten the conversation around the table by commenting on how delicious the soup was.

Rachel stood to clear the soup bowls and bring the main course to the table. Maxine rose to help, and when she got into the kitchen, put the ultrasound picture back on the counter. "I'm sorry. I am so, so sorry. I didn't mean to cause problems. I just got excited at the prospect of a niece or nephew to spoil."

Rachel put her hand on Maxine's arm. "It was my fault. I was late and got discombobulated at seeing everyone here already that I didn't think to hide the ultrasound picture."

Rachel and Maxine worked as a team to serve the rest of the meal, clear the dishes, and serve the honey cake and coffee. The wine flowed freely, especially between Steve and his father. Rachel abstained. The atmosphere was tense; the conversation stilted. It veered from inconsequential talk to local politics, and to how the Cleveland Indians postseason playoffs were going. The fact that the Indians still had a chance to win the Pennant was the most animated conversation of the evening. The two elephants playing in the corner were Rachel's pregnancy and Miriam's rapid decline.

Everyone was ready to leave earlier than usual, and Rachel, in her exhaustion, was glad to see them go. They thanked her for the scrumptious meal. She hugged Steve's family and again wished them all Shanah Tovah Umetukah 'Have a good and sweet year.' As they hugged, Miriam whispered into Rachel's ear, "You'll make the right decision. You have a good head on your shoulders."

Rachel gave Maxine a longer than usual hug and thanked her for all her help.

- Chapter 29 -

After everyone left, Rachel asked Steve to help her finish clearing the table and get the pots and pans soaking. As Rachel carried dessert dishes into the kitchen, Steve followed her empty-handed and shoved her roughly against the counter by the sink. The china fell out of her hands, clattering everywhere. One dish crashed in pieces on the floor. Rachel yelled. Her hip hurt where he had slammed her into the counter.

Stunned, she swirled around with tears in her eyes.

Steve shouted, "What the fuck…what a devious way to announce to my family that you are pregnant! What the hell were you thinking?"

"When Maxine found the ultrasound on the counter, she ran out to make the announcement before I could stop her."

Steve slapped Rachel's face. "Don't go blaming my little sister. You're the idiot that got pregnant."

Rachel held her cheek and yelled, "Don't you ever hit me again!"

"You deserved it."

At that, Rachel gave Steve a quick kick in the groin, thankful for the years of playing soccer. He doubled over and yelped in pain. She pushed past him and ran out the door. She ran and ran and ran, tears blinding her. Panting, with a pain in her side, she came to their synagogue where the Rosh Hashanah services had already started. She wiped her eyes, walked in, picked up a program, and sat on the back pew, hoping to remain hidden. On the right side of the Bimah, the cantor led the congregation in songs welcoming the holiday, songs familiar and comforting to her. The lights were dim, and she felt safe and hidden as she caught her breath, listened to the prayers, and attempted to pray.

The congregation prayed together, "May the One who causes peace to reign in the high heavens let peace descend on us, on all Israel, and all the world."

The rabbi said, "Those who have made peace in their house, it is as though they have brought peace to all of Israel, indeed to all the world. Peace will remain a distant vision until we do the work of peace ourselves."

Rachel listened. *I don't think I can make peace with Steve. I'm not sure he wants peace with me.* She left the service early, sneaking out the back door. She wanted to avoid familiar faces and probing questions.

A cold drizzle started. "What do I do now? I can't go home." Rachel wandered around the dark suburban streets, trying to avoid streetlight spotlights. She found herself on her mother's street. The lights were still on, so she knocked, and her mother answered. Rachel saw her mother's new boyfriend sitting in the background at the dining room table. The candles were lit, and two wine glasses were half full. Rachel waved at him and said, "L'Shana Tovah." He waved back.

Her mother hissed, "What are you doing here?" Her mother didn't invite her in, nor did she notice that Rachel was shivering.

Rachel tried to hold back her tears. It was too painful to expose any weakness or vulnerability to her mother. Through her tears, she mumbled, "Steve pushed and slapped me."

"I'm sure you deserved it. You need to see a shrink."

Rachel inhaled deeply, wiped her eyes on her sleeve, and mumbled, "Sorry to bother you. L'Shana Tovah." She turned away from her mother and walked down the front steps as her mother shut the door behind her.

The cold drizzle matured into a bone-chilling rain. Rachel turned her face up to the black weeping sky to wash away the tears. Her tears flowed from a deep, dark abyss of infinite pain. She berated herself for thinking that it was a good idea to stop by her mother's. Her mother had a knack for making her feel despicable. She had seen psychologists before, and they always gave her the same advice; stop seeking love from her mother, who was incapable of giving it. It occurred to her for the first time that maybe she had fallen into the same pattern with Steve. She wondered where she could go without her car, wallet, and cell phone, especially on Rosh Hashanah Eve when all her acquaintances were celebrating.

She headed in the direction of Elizabeth's house, a few miles away. She shivered as she trudged along in the dark, cold rain. An hour later, warm lights emanating from Elizabeth's living room and front porch beckoned Rachel to knock on the door.

Elizabeth opened the door to find Rachel, soaking wet, teeth chattering, shivering and weeping. She put her arms around her and said, "You look worse than anything the cat ever dragged in."

Elizabeth held Rachel as she stood in the front foyer weeping and dripping water. She then abruptly ordered her, "Take your sopping clothes off and I'll find you something dry." She handed her a towel before hunting for dry clothes.

Rachel obediently disrobed, dropping her wet clothes on the foyer floor. Elizabeth returned with a sweatshirt, sweatpants, and a warm blanket. "I'm afraid my clothes might be a little baggy on you. You might have to hold them up with one hand like Marguerite."

Elizabeth wrapped Rachel in the blanket, led her to the couch, held her in her arms and ran her fingers through Rachel's long, wet, curly hair as she cried on and off. "I left the lights on for you. Your fiancé Steve found my number in your phone and called a few hours ago. He said that you were acting crazy and wandered out of your house."

"He told you that? I may be crazy, but I didn't wander out of the house; I ran. He blamed me for becoming pregnant and told me to get an abortion. Tonight, he shoved me into the counter and slapped me." She began weeping again.

Elizabeth just held her in her arms, rubbing her back. "Do you want me to call Steve to let him know you're safe?"

"No. I don't want him to know where I am. Definitely don't want to see him."

Elizabeth nodded. "Stay here tonight. I have two spare bedrooms with clean sheets on both beds."

Rachel looked into Elizabeth's eyes. "Thank you. I am so tired, thank you. Somehow, I knew your home would be a safe place. Are you sure I won't be a bother?"

"Bother? Your landing on my doorstep added excitement to my otherwise dreary existence. Are you hungry? Can I get you a cup of tea?"

"I'm not hungry, but I could use a cup of hot tea."

As they sipped the tea with honey, Rachel said, "Thanks, I couldn't go back home tonight."

"You're damn right you're not going back. Don't ever return to that son of a bitch. You deserve so much better. You can stay here for as long as you need."

"My life is a shambles. I don't know what the next step is. Steve has a court case tomorrow. It's Rosh Hashanah but he's only observant when it's convenient. I'm hoping that while he's at court, I can pick up my car, cell phone, laptop, clothes, and a few other belongings."

Elizabeth knitted her brow. "What if he's around? Will you feel safe? Do you want me to go with you just in case? I can get off work early to help you."

"Thanks. I could use your help. I am hoping to go to a Rosh Hashanah service in the morning. I've never missed one in my life. I'm hoping that Steve will still be at court during the afternoon, and we can pick up my stuff without my having to deal with him. Services usually end by noon, and then I'll start looking for apartments."

"Don't rush into looking for an apartment. You can stay here for as long as you need."

When they finished their tea, Elizabeth gave her the choice of either Becky or Lauren's old bedroom. Becky's bedroom shouted from the hall with boisterous mismatched colors of orange, red, and purple, whereas Lauren's bedroom was the picture of calmness and peace with blue walls and a pale green comforter. Rachel chose Lauren's room.

Elizabeth smiled. "That's the room I'd pick for myself. Becky loved noisy clashing colors even as a baby." Elizabeth showed Rachel where the bathroom was and handed her a fresh towel and washcloth.

When Elizabeth closed the door behind her, Rachel slid between the crisp sheets and pulled the comforter to her neck. The minute her head hit the pillow, she sunk into a bewildering dreamland. She dreamt that Darnell kicked Steve. Then she searched for a little girl lost and wandering. In another dream, Ms. Leggett yelled at her for getting wet in the rain.

When she awoke the following morning, it took her a few minutes to figure out where she was. Then, with a shudder, she remembered the previous night and slid back under the covers.

Rachel eventually pulled herself out of bed. Eli had hung her dry clothes on the doorknob. Rachel took a shower, letting the hot water massage her back and neck. The clothes hanging on the doorknob were the 'school marm' outfit for the Rosh Hashanah dinner the night before. Perfect for attending synagogue services. However, she wished for clean underwear.

She wandered downstairs. Eli had left her a long note detailing the food options in the refrigerator, a pot of hot coffee, and her laptop on the table with the password. Rachel discovered a jacket draped on the kitchen chair with a note pinned to it stating it was Lauren's jacket and she may need it today because the weather forecast is predicting a high of fifty degrees. Rachel marveled at Eli's kindness and hospitality as she ate yogurt with berries and sat down to enjoy her coffee. She turned on Elizabeth's laptop to search for a synagogue within walking distance. Many synagogues require admission tickets to high holy day services, but most never check and everyone is welcomed. She also knew that many Jewish people only attend services on the High Holy days so her presence at almost any synagogue today would go unnoticed. She didn't want to go to her synagogue because she didn't want to have to explain anything to anyone. She preferred to stay anonymous.

She looked forward to the sounding of the Shofar, heralding the beginning of the Days of Awe. When she was a child, the Shofar woke her up during a boring service. As she grew older, the sounding of the Shofar woke her from the mundane in her daily life, opening her heart to the mystery of God and this one life she was living.

- Chapter 30 -

The rain had stopped overnight, and the sun beamed in a blue sky. The leaves on the trees glistened with droplets, tears sparkling in the sun. Rachel walked to the synagogue in the cool air, grateful for Lauren's jacket. She arrived early, but several people were already milling around. She didn't have a ticket but walked in with the authority of one who had been there for years and knew her way around. She smiled amiably at the ushers as she found a side aisle seat towards the back.

The synagogue was standard as far as synagogues went. The Ark was front and center on the Bimah. A beautiful lamp hung from the ceiling in front of the ark. Candelabra framed the Ark on each side. Rachel watched a congregation of strangers' faces filing in. Even though she didn't recognize the faces, the congregation felt familiar. There was a low murmur of voices as people greeted one another. Men wore yarmulkas, and many women covered their heads with a variety of head coverings. Young families corralled rambunctious children running up and down the aisle. Occasionally a grandparent or two was part of the family group. She watched a young father carrying his toddler daughter on his hip down the aisle. Elderly people hobbled down the aisle, sometimes with a cane, a walker, or a younger person supporting them. Young couples sat close together, holding hands; older married couples sat comfortably apart, mostly conversing with their neighbors on either side.

Rachel read a few meditations before the service. She prayed with her whole heart for wisdom and guidance. She had two questions to ask God. Should she get an abortion? And should she leave Steve? Perhaps it was just two sides of the same question. Maybe she already knew the answers in her heart.

She remembered the four-hour abortion seminar in nursing school and the many impassioned and divisive arguments among her classmates. The main point of contention was the question of when the soul enters the embryo. The Evangelical Christian and Catholic students insisted that the soul entered the embryo the moment of conception, rendering abortion an act of murder. Rachel marveled that they could state with absolute certainty God's opinion on something that couldn't be measured or scientifically proven.

Since she was the only Jewish student in the class, her role was to present the Jewish arguments pro and con. In her research she discovered that there was no 'one' Jewish position. The name Israel means 'one who contends with God.' In Judaism, people don't just contend with God, but with each other. The Talmud and the Mishnah are voluminous commentaries arguing, and generally not agreeing, on the meanings of the various scriptures. There is never just one meaning or interpretation. Judaism is a religion comfortable with nuance and mystery.

She remembered her presentation to her fellow students. In her research she discovered that the Torah is remarkably silent on abortion, even though abortion in some form or another has existed throughout history in all cultures, though not as safe as it is now. The only scripture she could find remotely approaching the subject was Exodus 21:22. In that scripture, if two men are fighting and injure a pregnant woman accidentally so that she miscarries, the penalty is a fine. Not a big deal. Not murder. In many Talmudic texts, the fetus is considered a part of a woman's body until it can live on its own. The pregnant mother's life takes precedence over the fetus; an existing life takes priority over a potential life. This is especially true if there are health issues, mental pain, and in cases of infidelity, rape, and incest. As far as the issue of when the soul enters the fetus, some interpretations believe it happens with the infant's first breath, because of the quote in Genesis (2:7) where God formed man from the dust of the ground and then breathed life into his nostrils and the man became a living soul. The soul is peculiarly connected to the breath in Judaism.

She listened to the service and to her heart. It occurred to her that all the arguments in the Talmud were made by men. She remembered Miriam insisting that this was her decision. She wondered what the arguments would be if women wrote the Talmud. Then she questioned why, even to this current day, men are making the laws and decisions about women's pregnancies.

She listened intently. Many of the meditations in a Rosh Hashanah service are a celebration of life and a plea for its continuance. She read the words, "Therefore, choose life," knowing that reverence for life is one of the highest principles in Judaism.

At one point in the service the congregation read the ancient poem called the Unetanah Tokef. In a service honoring life, it's a poem describing the many ways a person can die. No one knows the author, but it's been included in Rosh Hashanah services since the Middle Ages. As she listened to the poem, her mind wandered to her own life and its many unanswered questions.

*"On Rosh Hashanah it is written, on the fast of Yom Kippur
this is sealed.
How many will pass away from this world.
How many will be born into it;
Who will live and who will die;
Who will reach the ripeness of age,
Who will be taken before their time;
Who by fire and who by water;
Who by war and who by beast;
Who by famine and who by drought;
Who by earthquake and who by plague:
Who by strangling and who by stoning;
Who will rest and who will wander;
Who will be tranquil and who will be troubled;
Who will be calm and who tormented;
Who will live in poverty and who in prosperity;
Who will be humbled and who exalted."*

Rachel wondered about this focus on death. She surmised that the specter of death is included in the service to remind people of life's fragility and preciousness. She considered the question of God deciding who shall live and who shall die. She thought of Steve's mother, Miriam, and worried it would soon be her time to go. She considered her dialysis patients. Did Harriet decide the time of her death when she withdrew from dialysis or did God? She thought of Ethel and her heart ached for how she had died from blood loss on dialysis.

She remembered sitting next to her father during Rosh Hashanah services. He was the one who taught her to love the sounding of the Shofar. But then came the Rosh Hashanah service the year he died, when he was no longer written in the Book of Life. That year, she cried at the blast of the Shofar and kept asking God why her father couldn't be one to have lived to see ripe age. Tears always came to her eyes when she thought of her father.

She asked God if she should abort the pregnancy. To abort was the rational, logical decision; she wasn't prepared to be a single mom, finances would be tight, and the child wouldn't have a father figure. That's what her brain told her, but her heart remembered the tiny fetus swimming in her womb. She decided to give the life growing within her a chance at life. It was an act of faith in God and in life, especially during these holy days when the Book of Life was open. She had a sense that with this choice, she had become the author of the book of her own life for the first time. Before today, the book of her life had been written by others who told her who she was and how she was supposed to live.

Rachel watched the two restless, squiggly small children in the row in front of her. The little girl pinched her older brother. He squawked and made a face as the mother shushed them both. A few seats down, a mother held a contented baby, making pleasant baby noises. Another mother carried a crying baby out of the synagogue. *That will be me this time next year.*

If she kept the pregnancy, the question of leaving Steve became moot. Life with him had become lonely and unsatisfying even before he pushed and slapped her. If she left him, money would be tight. Perhaps it was the prospect of financial security that kept her with him for so long? She felt vulnerable and exposed when she imagined the road ahead as a single mother.

Then came the long, mournful blasts from the Shofar. Today the Shofar blast was a plaintive cry from her wide-awake heart for help and strength.

She returned to Elizabeth's house after the service, made herself a peanut butter and jelly sandwich, and fell asleep on the couch.

- Chapter 31 -

Elizabeth woke Rachel with a gentle touch. "Wake up little rosebud. It's time for our foray to gather your belongings."

Rachel stretched, yawned, and sat up. "I'm looking forward to clean underwear."

Elizabeth asked, "How was church, er, I mean synagogue?"

"I decided to keep the pregnancy."

"That choice was taken from you today. The Heartbeat Law went into effect today, essentially banning abortion before most women even know they are pregnant."

"You mean I did all that soul-searching for nothing?"

"Yup. Your choices don't matter." She shook her head. "The law is nonsensical. The Republicans at the statehouse think that an electrical current between some cells, amplified and augmented by an ultrasound machine to mimic the sound of a heartbeat, means there is a beating heart. A six-week-old embryo doesn't have a heart to beat yet."

Rachel sighed and shook her head. "Whoever is making these decisions doesn't know what the real world is like. When I was in nursing school, I assisted with an abortion for an eleven-year-old girl raped by her uncle. She had just entered puberty…no real breasts, scant pubic hair. She was still a child."

Elizabeth nodded. "When I was a teenager, right before Roe-vs-Wade, one of my friends died from a self-induced abortion. I still wonder what her life could have been. I never imagined we'd return to those awful days."

As they headed out the door, Elizabeth stopped. "Shall I bring my gun?"

Rachel did a double take. "You have a gun?"

Elizabeth laughed. "I do have a gun, but I was just kidding about bringing it. My daughters bought it for me after Ebony died. They worry about me living alone without a barking dog to scare an intruder. They should be more concerned about me having a gun in the house. I don't know how to use it… not even sure if I can point it in the right direction." Elizabeth smirked. "I suppose I could bring it without any bullets and wave it around to scare Steve."

"I'm not afraid of Steve hurting me physically, just afraid of what we might say to each other."

"He slapped you and shoved you into the counter. That sounds physical to me."

"I can defend myself…I kicked him in the nuts."

"I suspect he has also been verbally abusive towards you."

Rachel scrunched her face. "Not abusive per se, just critical and controlling."

As they walked to the car, Elizabeth asked, "Do you have a key to get into your house?"

"We hide a key under an empty flowerpot in the garage."

They pulled into the driveway. Rachel's car was still parked in the turnaround where she had rushed into the Rosh Hashanah dinner the evening before, a lifetime ago. Rachel was hopeful for a moment, thinking that perhaps she had left her keys in the car. She tried the car door, which was locked and noticed her purse and cellphone on the passenger seat.

The key under the flowerpot had disappeared. Rachel and Elizabeth worked as a team, looking under anything that could be picked up or moved, including the lawnmower, garbage cans, recycle containers, old paint cans, charcoal bags, the grill, fertilizer bags, and odd yard tools. Finally, the two women stood together looking out from the garage at the back entrance of her house, admitting defeat.

Elizabeth, hands on hips, looked at Rachel. "What's Plan B?"

Rachel pointed to the milk chute. "Maybe I can crawl into

the milk chute? I used to do that growing up when my mom locked me out of the house."

Elizabeth laughed. "Rachel, you may be skinny, but I'd hate to have to call the fire department to get you unstuck from the milk chute. Let's check all the windows and doors." Everything was locked tightly on the first floor, but Rachel noticed an upstairs window opened a crack with a rose trellis leading to the window. She pointed to the window and the trellis and smiled.

Elizabeth shook her head. "Not a good idea. You're not dressed for that with your skirt and dainty shoes. Let's just call Steve to let us in."

"Let me just try. You can spot me at the bottom as I climb." Rachel started climbing the trellis as Elizabeth leaned her weight against the bottom, holding it against the house. Rose thorns pricked and scratched Rachel as she climbed. As she neared the top, ready to grab the windowsill, the trellis tore away from the siding. Rachel's feet slid off a rung, leaving her hanging on for dear life to the top rung. The trellis leaned at a forty-five-degree angle; Rachel's body swayed as her skirt fluttered in the breeze. "Uh-oh, you were right Eli. This was a stupid idea."

Elizabeth tried to push the trellis back against the house. "Can you jump?"

"My shoe just fell off. I'm afraid of hurting my foot. I'm such a klutz."

Just then Steve pulled into the driveway. His BMW screeched to a halt as he jumped out of his car and yelled, "What the fuck are you two doing?"

Rachel looked down at Elizabeth. "This may be awkward."

Steve ran to Rachel, grabbed her legs, and then her hips as he slowly lowered her to the ground. He moaned, complaining that his groin hurt.

Meanwhile, Elizabeth scooted away from the trellis so it

wouldn't knock her on the head as it crashed to the ground. Rachel found her shoe and slipped it on her foot.

Steve asked again. "What were you two doing?"

"The key under the flowerpot is gone. I'm taking my things."

"Taking your things? Why?"

She looked at the ground and kicked a broken rose with her toe. "I'm moving out."

Steve moved toward her. "Rachel, you can't just walk away. I promise I won't hit you ever again."

Rachel moved away from his touch. "Steve meet Eli, the NP that I work with."

Steve said quietly. "Thank you for your kindness when I called last night." He tilted his head and gave a knowing glance at the trellis on the ground. "I know you share my concerns."

Elizabeth shook her head. "I'll admit things look crazy, but Rachel is completely sane."

Steve replied, "Thanks for bringing her home. I can handle things from here."

Elizabeth put her arm over Rachel's shoulder. "I'm helping gather her belongings."

Rachel said, "I'm keeping the pregnancy. Once I find an apartment, I'll be back to pick up some kitchen items and furniture."

Steve frowned. "Don't expect me to pay for that fetus you insist on keeping."

"Even I know that's not how the law works. Besides, abortion isn't available in Ohio after today."

"I'll drive you to New York this weekend."

Rachel raised her voice: "I'm not getting an abortion. Are you going to let me in the house or not?"

Steve sighed and let them in the front door before sitting on the couch, arms folded across his chest.

Rachel glanced into the kitchen and saw that he hadn't cleaned up after the previous night's feast. She frowned when she saw the leftovers from yesterday's labors languishing in serving dishes, dry and unappetizing. Shards from the broken china were still scattered on the floor. A wave of sadness and loss washed over her. She grabbed the ultrasound picture and pre-natal vitamin prescription on the counter, before dashing upstairs to their bedroom, opening drawers and closets, gathering clothes and underwear. She left her cocktail dress and other fancy outfits that she wouldn't need, nor be able to fit into any time soon. She gathered her nursing books and journals. She grabbed her laptop, work keys, and stethoscope; the basics to get by. She ignored the expensive tchotchkes adorning the dressers but grabbed her old teddy bear out of the closet.

Elizabeth helped haul her stuff down the stairs and out the door. They stuffed Elizabeth's car but needed the space in Rachel's car for the rest. Her car was still locked, so she went to the living room and asked Steve for her car keys.

He shook his head. "I don't have them. You should know where you put them last. You lose everything."

Rachel raised her voice: "I know you have them! You used the phone in my car last night to call my friends and then locked my car door."

He reached into his pocket and threw her keys on the carpet in front of him.

She picked them up and slid them into her skirt pocket. Before turning to leave, she said, "I bet you also have the flowerpot house key."

He reached back into his pocket and threw it on the floor.

"One more thing. You need to move your car so we can get out of the driveway. I would hate to ruin the lawn driving around your car." She shrugged. "What would the neighbors think?" Steve huffed and stood to move his car.

Rachel hurried out the back door, piled the rest of her belongings into the trunk and back seat, and slid into her car. She checked her purse to be certain that her wallet and charge cards were intact. Then she checked her phone, wondering how many calls Steve had made the previous evening. He had only called Eli, her mother, and her best friend Shelly. She gave a thumbs up to Elizabeth, who was sitting in her car, engine running. She turned on the ignition, and they drove out the driveway, past the broken trellis on the front yard with branches, leaves, and rose petals scattered everywhere.

It took them less than an hour to unload Rachel's belongings. When they finished, they collapsed on the living room furniture, sprawled with outstretched limbs.

"Thanks for helping me schlep all my stuff to your house. I couldn't have done it without you."

"I have your back."

Rachel started crying softly. "I can't believe it's over. For so many years I adored him. I don't know if he changed or if I changed. I kidded myself believing that we could make a life together. This pregnancy has opened my eyes to the whole picture. I kept trying to make myself into the person he thought I should be."

Elizabeth nodded. "He was full of promises today. Many women would have changed their minds and stayed, especially with his good looks and money."

Rachel sat quietly for a while before shaking her head. "He wanted you to think I'm crazy."

Elizabeth laughed. "I don't think you're crazy. I know you're crazy."

"I'm going to miss his family. His sister and I are friends, and his mother is so kind. I'm not sure I'll feel comfortable just showing up at their back door like I have for most of my life. Their home was my real home growing up."

They were quiet for a while until Rachel spoke, "I want to

make a dent in my school loans before the baby comes along. I think I'll take a part-time job as a home infusion nurse. Shelly, my best friend, has been trying to recruit me for months for her home infusion company, tempting me with good pay and good hours. I'll call her tomorrow. I'll also start looking for an apartment."

"Like I told you last night…no rush to move out. You can stay here and save your money. The past twenty-four hours have brought me more adventure than I've seen in years."

The following day, Rachel called Shelly, who was delighted that she would be working for her. They made plans for her orientation the following week on her day off from the dialysis unit. Her friend bent over backward to make things convenient for her.

Rachel continued working in the dialysis unit. She found the busy routine to be a welcome distraction from the upheaval in her personal life, and her anxieties about becoming a single mother. One day while Rachel assessed Darnell before he started dialysis she said, "Darnell, let me check your new fistula. I think we may be able to start using it next dialysis."

He held out his right arm for her to examine. She took it gently into her hand, palpated the vessel and listened to the bruit with her stethoscope. "It's looking good. I'll get an order to start using it on Monday."

J.R. glanced over. "The fistula might be okay, but your poor lady hasn't grown back her boob, leg, and arm."

Darnell shook his head, "The permcath is cool. No needles; so easy and painless. I'd be happy to wait a few more weeks or months. Maybe my lady needs a little more time…"

"Absolutely not Darnell. We call a permcath the 'white tube of death.' The tip of that plastic tube is in the right atrium of your heart. Bacteria love making little colonies on any foreign body. I've seen patients get infections in their joints, heart valves, and spinal cords from permcaths. The sooner we remove it the better."

Darnell nodded and spoke tenderly to the disfigured lady on his arm. "Honey, first they replaced your appendages with a large ugly scar, and now they want to stick big needles into your stomach and head. They are so mean around here."

- Chapter 32 -

Darnell loved Mama's Sunday dinners. Sundays were non-dialysis days and Mama always cooked a feast. In addition to Mama's cooking, Darnell loved roughhousing with his nephews while Mama put the finishing touches on the dinner. Last week they played football. The twins took turns with one of them being the football under Darnell's arm and the other playing the fullback trying to tackle him. Other Sundays they played basketball using the rusty net-less hoop that Darnell and Will played on growing up. Darnell would lift each of his two nephews close to the metal basket so they could drop the basketball into the hoop. He taught them how to dribble; sometimes pretending to dribble his nephews. Whatever the game, it was accompanied by a constant refrain of "Do it again, do it again!"

Today the two little boys climbed the old apple tree in the backyard. After each climbed to the second branch, Darnell would exclaim at how high they climbed, and how strong and amazing they were. As they held out their arms and jumped, he would catch them and twirl them around before putting them on the ground.

Mama called everyone in for dinner. Clarence and Lester never wanted to stop playing with Darnell, so they toddled, heads down as they followed their Uncle Dewy into the house. Darnell held them, one at a time, at the sink, put soap on their little hands, and made sure they washed and dried their hands before sitting down to eat, one on each side of him.

Mama had prepared pork fricassee, collard greens, creamed corn, and tomato casserole. Tomato casserole wasn't exactly a preferred item for a dialysis diet, but Darnell and J.R. were convinced that whatever food Mama made, just because she made it, couldn't possibly cause any harm.

Darnell experienced a slight headache, and his appetite wasn't as robust as usual. He chalked it up as one of the many inconveniences of being a dialysis patient.

They gathered around the table as Mama led the prayer. She prayed for Will in jail, mentioning that it was a dangerous place. She prayed that Darnell would be able to pawn his motorcycle to pay the bail. Then she prayed for a transplant for Darnell, and for strength and favor for Shanita in her new job. She looked at the twins on either side of Darnell, smiled at them, and prayed that they would grow in wisdom, knowledge, and strength like Jesus. While she prayed for them, Darnell put a hand on each of their heads. He didn't want his bad attitude towards God to block any blessings that might be headed their way. Finally, Mama looked at J.R. and thanked God for bringing him back into her life. J.R. thanked God for letting him be a part of this wonderful family after so many years of living alone.

Darnell didn't want Mama to think he was being totally selfish in waiting until November to pawn his motorcycle, so when she finished praying, he reminded her again, for the hundredth time, his belief that Will was safer in jail rather than out running with the unsavory characters with guns that he was hanging with. He also reminded Mama that he really couldn't pawn the motorcycle until November. "Will's court date isn't until February. If I don't return the money the pawn shop gives me within four months, they can sell my bike."

Shanita smiled at Darnell. "Darnell loves riding his motorcycle most when the autumn leaves start to fall. It's his favorite time of year."

Darnell returned her smile. "Shanita, did I ever tell you that you are my favorite sister, and, on top of that, the best one?"

Mama looked at Darnell. "I know it seems to you that I love Will more than I love you because I worry so much about him. It's just that I know you're going to be okay. Someday you'll receive a transplant and get off dialysis. I went to the transplant office a few months back to see if I could give you one of my kidneys, and they told me to lose forty pounds."

Shanita added another scoop of tomato casserole to her plate. "That's even worse than the thirty pounds they told me I had to lose."

J.R. leaned towards Darnell, elbows on the table. "I'm the perfect weight. Would you like one of my kidneys?"

Everyone looked at him and groaned.

One of Ruby's supreme desires was to have her entire family attend Sunday church services with her. She reveled in the fact that J.R. had started attending with her every Sunday but still wanted her grandchildren to attend. She asked Darnell, "When are you coming to church with me and J.R.?"

Shanita waved her fork. "I remember you ushering Darnell and Will out of church every Sunday for misbehaving."

Mama chuckled. "And they'd both be beseeching the congregation to pray for them as I dragged them out."

Darnell became serious. "God and I aren't on the best of terms these days. I'm afraid I might bump into Him in church and say something I regret later."

Mama replied, "Ain't nothing that you can say to God that God don't already know. Come and listen to J.R. singing in the choir with me. His baritone voice has elevated our music to a new level."

Darnell grinned at J.R. "Perhaps J.R. will give us a concert in the dialysis unit."

J.R. grinned back at him, squinting his eyes to tell Darnell to shut up. They were remembering a dialysis session a few weeks earlier when Darnell had goaded J.R. into performing his choir repertoire. J.R.'s off-key singing had several patients laughing hysterically, but several others missed the peace and quiet of the buzzing dialysis alarms. The dialysis unit social worker intervened, telling J.R. to cease and desist his concert or else find another dialysis unit. Since that day, patients and staff razzed J.R. about his singing; one patient reported hearing a screech owl the previous night and thought for a minute it was J.R. serenading her outside; another patient suggested that a recording of his singing might be better than a cattle prod in getting him to jump out of bed in the morning; the unit secretary suggested that the Division of Natural Resources might be interested in using his singing skills as a moose mating call. Others requested a copy of his dialysis concert schedule so they would be forewarned to skip dialysis that day.

Ruby, not privy to the dialysis singing adventure remarked, "That's a wonderful idea. I'm sure everyone in the unit will be blessed."

Darnell and J.R. howled with laughter.

Later, J.R. took Darnell aside and said quietly, "I know my singing isn't anything that would bring you to church. I can't explain it, but when I'm singing in the choir, everything that is painful and disconnected in my life dissolves. I don't feel so alone. We suffer together. I feel held by God. I hope you come sometime not for my singing, but for the fellowship."

The rest of the meal was a companionable affair. Lester and Clarence had a thousand questions of why this and why that. Since Mama had prayed that they grow up to be like Jesus, Lester asked Mama about Jesus. Mama delighted in telling her great-grandchildren stories about who Jesus was. Clarence said he didn't want to grow up to be like Jesus, he wanted to grow up to be like Uncle Derry, and Lester nodded in agreement.

J.R. regaled the gathering with stories of being a school bus driver back in the day. As Darnell listened to J.R.'s stories, he wondered if he should be more amazed that the students survived J.R. or that J.R. survived the students.

Shanita announced that she had been at her job for six months and was now eligible for tuition reimbursement to go to school. She reported that the NP who rounded at the nursing home told her that she had started at that very nursing home as a nurse's aide and, with tuition reimbursement over the years, continued school every semester for ten years, going from an LPN to an RN and finally to the NP she was now. The NP had given her, her old stethoscope and blood pressure cuff. Everyone around the table told her that she would be the best nurse ever.

Chapter 33

After dinner, Darnell felt worse and decided to go home early. "I think I'm coming down with something." He drove Shanita and the twins home and they hugged at the entrance to the apartment building before heading to their separate apartments.

Shortly after settling into his apartment, Darnell suddenly felt dizzy, chilled, and weak. He collapsed on his couch and called Shanita. "Hey sis, something's wrong. I feel funny. Can you bring your new blood pressure cuff?"

Darnell had never made such a phone call, not even the time he lost all that blood on dialysis.

A minute later, Shanita was at his side with the twins, trying to take his blood pressure. She couldn't find it. First, she thought there was something wrong with the cuff, then she thought there was something wrong with her technique, but when she felt his cool, clammy skin and saw the beads of sweat on his forehead, she shook her head and moaned. "Oh no, he's in trouble." She called 911.

He didn't have the strength to object. As they waited for the ambulance, Shanita covered Darnell with a blanket and hovered over him, biting her lip and twisting her hair. The twins stood next to her, fretting and whining as they patted Darnell's stomach.

When the ambulance arrived, Shanita and the twins moved out of the way to give the EMTs room. The EMTs found an extremely low blood pressure and a very rapid heart rate. His oxygen level was low. They started an IV on him, gave him oxygen, put a heart monitor on him, and hoisted him onto the stretcher. Shanita strapped the twins into their car seats and followed the shrieking ambulance to the hospital.

The ER team worked feverishly to save him. They put him on a ventilator and put large IV lines in his larger vessels so they could give him enough fluid and medicine to get his blood pressure up. They took multiple blood cultures and tubes of blood before starting him on three potent antibiotics. They removed his dialysis catheter before transferring him to the ICU.

Shanita cried and bit her fingernails as she waited on the ICU waiting room couch. Her sons patted her arm and cuddled close to her. After a few hours the doctor came to the waiting room with an update. By this time, the twins were asleep on the couch, their heads on her lap. The doctor told Shanita that Darnell's body was in shock from a dangerous blood infection. His condition was grave, and the next few days would determine if he would survive. The doctor advised her to go home and get some rest. He promised to call with any news. The nurses allowed her and the twins to go to his ICU cubicle to say good night. Darnell was intubated and sedated and didn't know they were there. They all cried to see him like this. The twins kept saying, "Wake up Derry, wake up Derry." Shanita kissed Darnell on his forehead and said, "I love you. Did I ever tell you that you're my favorite brother?"

On the way home Shanita stopped at Mama's and told her and J.R. what happened. Mama was in her nightgown but got dressed immediately and told J.R., "We're going to the hospital for a prayer vigil." She called all her choir friends and asked for prayers.

The following morning, Shanita received a phone call from the ICU doctor. He told her that Darnell's vital signs were improving; the antibiotics were working. The crisis had passed. They were weaning him off the medications that kept his blood pressure up. They suspected that the dialysis catheter may have caused an infection in a valve in his heart, and they would be doing further testing in the coming days. He was still on a ventilator, but they were hopeful that they could start weaning him off in a day or so. He would receive dialysis today using the new fistula in his arm, hoping to avoid another catheter in his chest. He would remain hospitalized for at least two weeks.

Shanita asked the doctor to give the update to Mama in the waiting room. The doctor found Mama kneeling and praying next to the couch that J.R. slept on. When Mama heard that Darnell had turned the corner, she stood up, said, "Thank you Jesus," and woke J.R. to return home to sleep.

- Chapter 34 -

On Monday morning, when Rachel checked the hospitalization list, her stomach dropped when she learned of Darnell's admission to the ICU. A pit of anxiety concerning Darnell's welfare settled in her stomach, and she had a hard time concentrating on her work. When J.R. arrived on second shift, she pestered him with questions about what happened. He told Rachel the entire story of the dinner at Mama's and then Darnell's quick decline and admission to the ICU. He described Mama's prayer vigil in the waiting room.

Rachel was touched to hear that Darnell's mother spent the entire night praying for her son. She couldn't imagine her own mother praying for her for thirty seconds. She wondered what a person would say to God non-stop all night. How could anyone pray that long? She also wondered if it made a difference.

After work that day, Rachel stopped by the hospital to check on Darnell. She usually didn't visit her patients in the hospital but knew she wouldn't be able to sleep that night until she was sure he was going to be okay. She spoke with his nurse, who described how, for several hours, they thought they would lose him. She told Rachel that they were planning to start weaning him off the ventilator the following morning. Tears filled her eyes when she saw him on the ventilator. She studied his face, heart monitor and vital signs, before walking to his bedside and grabbing his hand. She whispered, "Darnell, I need you to stay alive. You're not allowed to die." She imagined his hand squeezing hers.

A few weeks rolled by. Rachel appeared the same on the

outside, but her interior landscape resembled a house in the aftermath of a tornado. She was pregnant and had walked away from her life trajectory with Steve. She felt untethered, a refugee from her previous life, dependent upon the kindness of her friends. Insecurities that she thought she had conquered bubbled to the surface. She felt weak and vulnerable, crying on a dime. She didn't miss Steve as much as she thought she would though. She missed Darnell. His vacant dialysis chair left an emptiness in her heart.

One day, while rounding, Rachel arrived at Marguerite's chair. "Since you returned a few weeks ago we've removed close to eight pounds of fluid, your blood pressure is back to normal, and the swelling in your feet is gone. How are things going with you?"

"I'm better. You all do a good job. I just didn't see it before because I hated dialysis, and everyone associated with it. Please sit a moment, I want to tell you the story."

Rachel looked around the unit, not having time to spare, but pulled up a chair and sat to listen.

Marguerite started her tale. "After my last dialysis here, we flew to Cancun and took a taxi to a shiny new hospital with glass windows. The nurses and doctors spoke to me in English, and I felt I was in good hands. We told the hospital staff, as instructed by our broker, that I had arrived to receive a kidney transplant from a relative. The surgery was successful, and the new kidney started making urine before they closed the incision.

The day after the surgery, except for the soreness over the incision, I felt better than I had felt in years. I had forgotten what normal felt like. They discharged me from the hospital two days later and gave me a three-month supply of anti-rejection pills and some pain pills for my incision.

My husband and I lounged around Cancun for a few weeks. Those weeks were heavenly; I peed like an ordinary human and ate every forbidden food: orange juice, tomatoes, avocados, potatoes, bananas, chocolate, and margaritas with salt coating the rim of the glass." Marguerite frowned. "I called the new kidney my little baby and every day patted it on my tummy."

Rachel glanced at her watch.

"A few weeks after returning to Cleveland, my feet started to swell and the incision over the new kidney hurt. When I developed fevers, I thought my new kidney was infected, so I made an appointment to see Dr. Burnouf. He told me my body was rejecting the kidney and admitted me to the hospital that day to salvage it. I spent weeks in the hospital as they tried every possible intervention.

"The soreness over my kidney became more painful as the days progressed. One afternoon they sent me to radiology for a scan. While waiting in the hallway for the procedure, I felt an excruciating pain in my stomach as the kidney ruptured. I died and arrived in a beautiful garden with a river running through it. The flowers waving in the breeze were more colors, shades, and hues than anything seen on earth. I didn't just see the colors, I felt them, heard them, and tasted them. People sang and danced. The music was magnificent, with sounds of water, wind, and drums. I didn't just hear the music; I felt its textures and saw its colors. I wanted to stay there forever."

Rachel interjected, "That sounds like a hallucination. It may have been from the anesthesia during the surgery to remove the kidney."

Marguerite shook her head. "I know I died. There was a big tree in the middle of the garden, and someone told me that if I could make it to the tree, I could stay. I ran as fast as I could to the tree, but a little, brown-skinned girl blocked my path. She took my hand and told me that I had to return to earth to make things right."

Marguerite's eyes filled with tears. "Dr. Burnouf told me

that the kidney they removed from me belonged to a small child… I think, no, I know, that the little girl who took my hand was my kidney donor. I kept calling the kidney my baby, and here it was the kidney of someone else's baby."

Rachel's eyes teared up, and she reached for Marguerite's hand.

"I thought my sufferings on dialysis were unbearable, but now I can't stop thinking about refugee children being kidnapped and their bodies destroyed for money. I'm trying to figure out how to make things right, like that little girl told me to do."

"What can you do? No one has been able to get rid of the cartels."

"I don't think I can get rid of the cartels, but I've heard of a little town in the state of Jalisco, on the shores of Lake Chapala, called San Pedro, which is considered the kidney disease capital of the world. Young people living there die of kidney disease in their twenties and thirties. No one knows the cause, but it may be that the water they drink and bathe in is toxic from the industries lining the river that feeds the lake. The people are afraid to drink the water, so they drink Coca-Cola instead."

Rachel shook her head. "Coke? Not a good choice for anyone with kidney problems. Maybe you can arrange for clean water to be delivered to them? Do you remember Richard, before he received the transplant? He delivered bottled water to the people in Flint, Michigan, every weekend with his truck."

Marguerite said, "I'd like to do something like that to start, but I'd also like to stop the pollution causing the poisoned water. It may take years of political wrangling and all my money, but I'll figure out something."

Rachel walked away from Marguerite, amazed at her transformation and wondering if the story of the little girl really happened. She also wondered about the doctors in the shiny hospital. What was their connection to the cartels?

She continued rounding and arrived at Joseph Fiorelli's chair (Anthony's father, Steve's colleague, who sought her advice at the cocktail party). At the time she had reassured Anthony that his dad would adjust to dialysis, but looking at him today, the alarm bells in her head went off. His clothes were disheveled, his hair unkempt, and he needed a shave. His body odor broadcasted that he hadn't showered for days.

He sat sullenly as she greeted him. "How are things going?"

"Fine."

She sat by his chair for a few moments saying nothing as she reviewed his chart. "You're losing weight and are starting to look a bit rugged."

"I'm losing weight because I can't eat anything."

"No appetite? Abdominal pain? Nausea and vomiting? Or are you finding the renal diet intolerable?"

A commotion at the door interrupted their conversation. Elizabeth walked into the unit with a lanky golden labradoodle on a leash. Eli and the dog were both smiling. Everybody oohed and aahed over the light brown fluffy giant teddy bear of a dog; patients in the waiting area, patients leaving the unit, the secretary, the techs…everyone.

Rachel asked, "Where'd you get the dog?"

The dog looked directly into Rachel's eyes, and she instinctively petted the dog's curly head.

"Buckeye's my new service dog. Just pretend he isn't here. My daughters brought him over this morning. He's a diabetic-alert dog and will pick up a scent when my blood sugar is too low or too high. He'll jump on me if my blood sugar drops. If I become unconscious, there is a device in my home where he can put his paw on to dial 911."

"How'd they get him? I googled diabetic alert dogs after Ebony died and learned that a diabetic alert dog can cost over twenty thousand dollars."

"My daughter Becky has connections. This dog's owner died last week."

"I hope the former owner didn't die of a low blood sugar reaction."

Elizabeth laughed. "Yeah, me too, but I'm already smitten with Buckeye. I wouldn't return him even if he's incompetent. Buckeye and I are scheduled for more personalized training this weekend."

Ms. Leggett heard all the commotion and sauntered into the unit. "Dogs aren't permitted in a dialysis unit."

"Martha, this is Buckeye, my new service dog. He will be accompanying me on my rounds starting tomorrow. You won't even know he's here."

"Everyone knows he's here. A person would have to be blind to miss that beast."

"Here are his papers. According to the ADA, he can be anywhere I need to be."

Martha waved aside the papers. "It's not just about you and your giant galoot. I have patients in this unit to protect. What if the machine alarms rile him up? What if a patient is allergic to or afraid of dogs? What if he has fleas? What about the germs he'll track in? I'm calling the regional director tomorrow. Buckeye needs to stay home when you're rounding." She walked away.

Rachel glanced at Buckeye, willing him to growl at Ms. Leggett, but he just wagged his tail.

Rachel returned to her rounding and the rest of the afternoon passed smoothly. That night she woke up in the middle of the night distressed when she remembered her unfinished conversation with Joe Fiorelli. "How could I have allowed myself to get so distracted?" She resolved to address his possible depression as soon as he arrived at the unit on Wednesday. As she considered Mr. Fiorelli, she pictured his seating arrangement in the dialysis unit. *Perhaps his chair assignment is the problem? What if I transferred his chair, so he sits to the left of J.R.? J.R. would make for a more entertaining dialysis session. Phil, the patient currently sitting to the left of J.R., always has his head in his laptop, oblivious to the dialysis unit milieu.*

Rachel often woke in the night thinking of her patients and many times remembering something she had forgotten to do. Usually, she would drift back to sleep, but tonight sleep eluded her. Her heart ached for Darnell on the ventilator with his infected heart valve.

- Chapter 35 -

Rachel's main goal the following Wednesday was to help Joe Fiorelli. She studied the dialysis schedule and determined that it would be easy to switch Phil and Joe's schedules and seating arrangements. Joe would now be seated next to J.R. Phil would start dialysis a half-hour earlier, Joe a half-hour later. She got the okay from Martha Leggett. Phil was delighted to get on the machine earlier, but Joe was disgruntled at the half-hour delay. His son Anthony approached Rachel with his displeasure with his father's later on time.

Rachel directed Anthony into the conference room to explain the plan outside the earshot of the patients. "I switched his seat. It's my fault. When I saw your father on Monday, I became worried about how depressed your dad seemed. I know you were concerned about his depression when we talked at the cocktail party, but lately, he seems to be getting worse, not better."

Anthony agreed. "I've tried everything I could think of to snap him out of it. I take my parents for outings every Sunday afternoon, but it's not helping."

Rachel listened. "Your dad will now be sitting next to J.R. He has a knack for bringing joy to the other patients in the unit. Until today, your father was sitting between a lady on one side who is a non-stop complainer, and, on the other side, a lady with dementia who hollers all the time. His seat assignment was in a very depressing neighborhood, so I switched him. I'm also going to ask Dr. Burnouf to evaluate him when he comes in for his rounds today. Sometimes he recommends counseling, sometimes he prescribes an antidepressant, sometimes both."

"I hope it works. He needs something."

She shrugged. "Me too. No guarantees. The only guarantee I can give you is to do the best we can to help your dad adjust."

Anthony leaned forward with his elbows on the conference table and lowered his voice, "I heard that you and Steve broke up."

"How did you find out so quickly?"

"For the past six months or so, there've been rumors of hanky-panky with his secretary. He came in to work a few weeks ago and announced that he left you. Now the two of them are openly together, all lovey-dovey. Disgusting."

Rachel frowned. "The first time I thought there was something between them was at the cocktail party. What's her name?" *That schmuck. All those months he was mean to me; he was fooling around. I should have kicked him in the balls harder.*

"Her name is Kathy, and she's a gold digger. She has already had a few affairs with other partners, but they don't last long."

Rachel was relieved to learn that the gossip at the office was that Steve left her for some floozy. A more palatable story than the complicated, shameful story of her accidental pregnancy, Steve wanting her to get an abortion, and abusing her.

Anthony leaned back in the chair. "Steve's a jerk. If there's anything I can do for you, or if you just need someone to talk to, here's my card. Maybe we can meet for coffee sometime?"

She thanked Anthony for the card and put it in her pocket.

Rachel returned to the dialysis unit in time to observe Joe starting dialysis in his new chair. J.R. was already asking Joe questions about electricity because Joe was an electrician. J.R. grinned and thanked Rachel for putting Joe next to him. Rachel smiled when she realized that J.R. assumed she had made the switch for his benefit. The previous week he had complained about his sessions dragging with Darnell in the hospital. There was no one to talk to. He had made several fruitless attempts to engage Phil in meaningful conversation, finally giving up. Mr. Freeman still occupied the corner chair, but it was difficult to carry on a conversation over an empty chair, especially with Mr. Freeman's hearing difficulties.

For the remainder of the shift, Rachel kept an eye on Joe and J.R.'s interactions. She purposely walked past them to eavesdrop on their conversations. J.R. instructed Joe on how to get used to dialysis life. He told him how hard it was for him in the beginning. Another time, as she passed their chairs, she heard J.R. tell Joe how to cheat on his diet by eating just a 'little bit' of the forbidden foods.

He told Joe that he eats whatever he wants before dialysis because the extra potassium and sodium are washed off with dialysis. "I have some great lunches before dialysis. Maybe someday we can meet for lunch together before coming here? We could meet at the Italian restaurant down the road. Occasionally I stop at the Chinese restaurant."

Rachel gave J.R. the evil eye with a shake of her head. "Now don't go teaching Joe all your bad habits in one afternoon. I should have known better than to put a new dialysis patient next to such a terrible influence."

Dr. Burnouf didn't show that day, so Rachel asked Elizabeth to see Joe. Elizabeth sat and spoke with Joe as he petted Buckeye.

At the end of the shift, Rachel asked Elizabeth if she had prescribed an antidepressant for Joe. Elizabeth shook her head. "It's easy to write a prescription, but so difficult to provide a cure. Our patients' medicine cabinets overflow with pills they don't take. Your idea to switch dialysis chairs was brilliant. J.R. and Joe seem to have hit it off and he seemed enamored of Buckeye. He's thinking of getting a dog now. Let's wait and observe how he does over the next few weeks."

- Chapter 36 -

Darnell improved by increments each day. His breathing tube came out the third day, and the following day he was able to get up and about slowly and gingerly. Physical therapy helped him regain his strength. Youth was on his side.

Shanita and her sons came every evening to visit him once he transferred to a regular floor. Seeing his nephews was the highlight of his day. Clarence and Lester would climb onto his hospital bed and play with the bed controls and the TV remote. J.R. and Mama came to visit also. On one of J.R.'s visits, Darnell asked J.R. to sing some of his choir repertoire to 'help improve his mood.' J.R. obliged, but the concert only lasted five minutes before a nurse arrived asking J.R. to be quiet because he was disturbing the other patients.

Darnell, amazed at how effective J.R.'s singing was in getting a nurse's attention, asked J.R. if he could stay with him for the remainder of his hospital visit. The nurse's call light was useless.

Throughout his hospitalization, Darnell remembered Rachel's visit. Sometimes he wondered if he had just hallucinated it. He kept hoping to see her face those long days in the hospital, but she never returned.

The blood infection had infected the tricuspid valve in his heart. To eradicate it he needed a six-week course of two different antibiotics. If the antibiotics didn't clear the infection, he'd need heart valve surgery. Once discharged, both antibiotics could be given in the dialysis unit, but one antibiotic needed to be administered IV at home on non-dialysis days.

Darnell arrived home after a three-week hospital stay. His

first morning back, he cleaned his apartment. He gazed at the cold downpour outside his window and Lake Erie's choppy steel waves and thought, *Even God is conspiring to help me clean this mess up.*

He started in his bedroom with four large garbage bags. He filled the bags with wrappers, empty soda cans, empty beer cans, mismatched worn socks, torn shirts, Will's glass pipe, and mementos from his old girlfriend. He discarded old term papers, wondering why he had saved them. He kept all his books though, organizing them with care on the bookshelf he constructed with bricks and boards. He discarded his nephews' broken toys, but the salvageable ones were put in a large wooden box with a lid that he had discovered in someone's garbage.

He wiped down surfaces, vacuumed, and dusted everything. He filled a bucket with soapy water and scrubbed the kitchen floor on his hands and knees. He had to change the water in the bucket a few times when it turned black. After spending the entire day cleaning, he stretched out on his couch for a nap, quite pleased with himself.

Shanita and the boys walked in later that evening as Darnell practiced his guitar.

Shanita looked around. "Oops, wrong place. This can't be your Uncle Derry's apartment."

Clarence and Lester jumped on his lap. They were getting bigger by the day and could no longer fit as easily as they had last year. He reached his arms around them and gave them a great bear hug until they started wriggling and screaming that he was squeezing them too tight. He showed them the toy chest. They were delighted to discover toys that they had forgotten. They grabbed a few cars and played together on the carpet.

Shanita inspected the apartment. "What inspired all this cleaning? I am witness to a miracle."

"I wanted you to be able to sit down and relax when you visit me, because you are my favorite sister."

"I don't believe that."

"You don't believe you're my favorite sister?"

"I don't believe you cleaned your pigsty for me."

"How about, the infusion nurse is coming the day after tomorrow to give me IV antibiotics, and I didn't want her to report me to the health department."

"I don't believe that either."

"How about I watched Marie Kondo on TV when I was in the hospital, and she inspired me."

"I don't believe that either."

"Well, here is the truth, so help me God, swear on the bible. Remember when I was unconscious, hovering between this life and the one beyond, and the doctors and nurses spent the entire night working on me, shocking my heart, performing CPR, and Mama was on her knees in the waiting room praying?

Shanita groaned and raised her voice, dragging out the words. "Of course, I remember all that, because I told you all that."

"Well, during those hours Jesus sat next to me on a park bench."

"I'm not sure I believe that either. Does Mama know?"

"Hell no. She'd drag me to church with all her homies and want me to stand in front of the congregation and tell them the story, with embellishment of course. This story is private, between me and Jesus, and now you, don't tell a soul."

"What did Jesus look like?"

He shrugged. "I don't know, I didn't really *see* Him."

"If you didn't see him, how did you know it was Him?"

"I just knew."

"What did He say to you?"

"He didn't say anything. I just felt loved."

"Now I know why you didn't want to tell Mama. She'd ask you all sorts of questions you can't answer. Did Jesus tell you to clean your apartment?"

"Nah, I cleaned it because it was dirty."

- Chapter 37 -

Two days later, on an indigo sky, Indian summer day, Darnell sat at his kitchen table, trying to catch up on his studies as he waited for the infusion nurse to arrive. The sliding doors to his balcony were open and the blue sky and leaves blowing in the breeze were a siren call to be out riding Rusty. The knowledge that he had been so close to death and was lucky to be alive made every second so much more precious.

He hated the thought of a visiting nurse coming four days a week for the next four weeks. *Such a waste of time.* He wondered if he could administer the antibiotics himself or maybe Shanita could help him with this chore.

He heard a knock at his door and opened it to discover Rachel standing there. His face exploded into a grin. He hugged her and beamed. "In my wildest dreams. I never expected to see you today. Why didn't you tell me in dialysis yesterday that you'd be here today?

Rachel smiled, backing off from his hug. "I didn't know you were on my schedule until this morning." She walked in and placed first a pad, and then her nurse's bag on the kitchen table. She had a light jacket over her lab coat and Darnell gently helped her remove it, their hands brushing and their eyes locking. Opera music played in the background. "Somehow, I don't picture you as an opera sort of guy."

"Well, I'm not really, but I have a paper that was due when I was in ICU comparing rap and opera. The professor is giving me until next Tuesday to finish it.

"And what have you discovered?"

"I don't know how people can call this shit music. It has no rhythm."

Rachel laughed. "And I don't know how people can call rap, music. It has no melody."

Darnell was in a party mood now. "I hope this infusion takes hours. Would you like a beer?"

Rachel laughed. "Do you really think I'd have a beer with you when I'm on the clock? The infusion usually takes about forty-five minutes."

"That isn't long enough. I'm sure I'm more complicated and will take more time than that. When did you become an infusion nurse?"

"I picked this job up to earn a few extra bucks."

"Why do you need a few extra bucks? I thought you were engaged to rich Steve Silverman, my lawyer, who hasn't been returning my phone calls."

"We broke up, and I'm hoping to make a dent in my school loans before the baby arrives."

He tilted his head, and his eyes narrowed. "What? Broke up? Baby arriving?" He sat at the kitchen table. "Tell me everything."

Rachel caught him up on the news.

"My sister is a single mom. You've chosen a difficult road."

"I know…I'm scared."

"Your ex is an idiot. I'm wondering if I should look for a smarter lawyer to take my case."

"He was a poor choice for a life partner, but he's a good lawyer…I think."

"I guess those are different skill sets. Do you miss him?"

"I miss the money and security, but I don't really miss *him*. Before we split, we lived parallel lives. We had stopped communicating or liking each other. I think of marriage as going through the fire together, but Steve wasn't willing to do the hard work. Steve wanted me to be someone I'm not."

Darnell, hopeful that maybe, after all, he might have a chance to win her heart, said, "I like you just the way you are."

He saw her face flush as she turned her attention to the job at hand.

"We've been talking way too long about me, but you're the one who almost died a few weeks ago. How are you feeling?"

"Feeling great with you sitting in my kitchen."

"No really. I need to know important things like your energy level, your appetite, if you are having any chest pain. Have you noticed any rashes or fatigue?"

"Physically, I'm feeling back to normal. All systems go, but just in case, you need to come and check on me every day, maybe twice a day, just to be sure…"

Rachel laughed. "Usually for home infusions, a catheter is placed in your arm or chest before discharge, and we use the catheter for the infusion. The doctors didn't want to risk another catheter in you with your recent sepsis and the heart valve infection, so we'll be inserting a butterfly needle into a vein in your arm every time and then removing it when the infusion is completed."

"Not a problem. I will love every minute you are here, four days a week for the next four weeks."

"I won't be here every time. Besides, we usually teach a family member or friend to do the infusions." She paused. "Doesn't your sister live in this building?"

"Shanita lives here but she works during the day, and needles make her squeamish. She can't do it. Couldn't you come after work? I know some days you get off early."

"It's not going to happen, even though I must admit, I looked forward to our visit today. I can't believe I'm getting paid to sit at your kitchen table."

Rachel washed her hands. "I don't remember your apartment being this clean the day I drove you home from dialysis. What happened? Did you hire a cleaning service?"

Darnell shifted a little. "Something happened to me when I was in the hospital."

Rachel sat at the kitchen table, plastic chair screeching against the floor. "Tell me."

"You can't tell anyone. The only other person who knows is my sister. The first night in the hospital, when I was in ICU, everyone thought I was dying. The staff worked all night to keep me alive, doing CPR and shocking my heart. I wasn't aware of any of that though. During that time, I sat on a park bench with Jesus. As He sat with me, I knew that my life mattered, even if I'm on dialysis and have no job. I'm where I need to be right now."

"Wow!" Rachel whispered softly.

"I've spent the past four years angry at God because I was stuck on dialysis without a future. God probably had to wait until I was unconscious for me to hear His side of the story."

Rachel tilted her head. "J.R. told me that Mama spent that night on her knees in the waiting room praying. I wonder if Jesus would have sat next to you if she had been home watching TV or sleeping?"

"I never thought of that. I wasn't planning on telling Mama, but maybe she needs to hear the story. I know she gets discouraged praying for me and my brother Will all the time."

"When I was in synagogue on Rosh Hashanah, I felt God tell me to keep this pregnancy. I think I would have liked to have Jesus, or any prophet, or teacher sit next to me in the pew. Do you think Jesus would ever come to a synagogue?"

"Jesus was Jewish. I bet he spent a lot of time teaching in synagogues. Maybe he was sitting next to you in the synagogue." He sat silently for a moment. "It might not be the location that matters so much as the state of our minds or hearts. I think I needed to be unconscious for God to break through to me."

Rachel started gathering her supplies. "Yeah, you might have a point there. Our thoughts and expectations can easily interfere with us hearing what God wants to tell us."

She checked Darnell's vital signs, listened to his heart and lungs, and checked his feet for any swelling and then examined his left arm for a good vein to place the tiny needle. His right arm was off-limits because of the new fistula. She pulled on rubber gloves. "Luckily, you continue to have some beautiful veins on your left arm despite the failed access."

"You find my veins beautiful?"

Rachel smiled.

As the antibiotics were infusing, Darnell asked, "When I was in ICU, I dreamt that you visited me. Did you really come?"

"I stopped by, just for a moment one day, on my way home from work."

"Why?"

"I was wondering how long you'd be in the hospital and if I could put another patient in your chair while you were away."

Darnell frowned. "I hoped that you visited me because you cared about me."

"Well, that too…I was worried."

"The entire time I was in the hospital, I kept looking at the door whenever anyone came, hoping to see your face."

Rachel looked into his eyes. "While you were watching an empty doorway, your empty chair in the dialysis unit caused a terrible ache in my heart."

"Do you have patients after me this afternoon?"

"You're my last patient. I saved the best for last."

"The weather outside today is exquisite. Come for a motorcycle ride with me. I have an extra helmet, and you can wear my leather jacket. I promise to keep you and the little one growing inside safe. There won't be many more days like today before the gray days arrive. I'll take you to some old growth woods. We can sit under the trees and watch the leaves fall."

"Watch the leaves fall? That sounds about as exciting as watching paint dry or waiting for water to boil."

"Apparently you've never watched leaves fall."

"Can't say that I have." Rachel stuttered and stumbled over her words. "I also promised Eli that I'd go for a walk with her and Buckeye when I got home today."

Darnell thought she was just making up an excuse but didn't want to let this moment pass. He laid his hand on Rachel's hand. "Call Eli and tell her that you can't make it."

Rachel was quiet for a few moments as the antibiotic solution dripped into Darnell's arm. She didn't say no. She didn't say yes. She focused on the open American History textbook on the kitchen table and flipped a few pages absently. Darnell hoped she was considering his proposition.

She looked up from flipping the pages. "Aren't you supposed to be studying? Don't you have midterms coming up?"

"I tried to study all day, but everything inside of me screams to get outside this afternoon."

"It isn't safe for you to be riding a motorcycle so soon after your hospitalization."

"I've ridden twice since I've been home. I had physical therapy when I was in the hospital and walked the halls every day. Motorcycle vibrations are healing to the human body."

Rachel pushed the hair out of her eyes. "I've always wanted to ride a motorcycle. But you need to promise that you will go slowly, and if I get scared, you'll bring me back."

Darnell, incredulous that she agreed to ride with him, shook her hand. "It's a deal."

"There is another more important promise that you need to make. You can't tell a single soul that you took me on your motorcycle, especially J.R. If he finds out, the world finds out, and I'll lose my job."

"Are you sure you want to risk your livelihood to ride a motorcycle with me? It doesn't seem like a particularly good, calculated risk." He hoped he wasn't discouraging her.

"Perhaps not, but this might be my one chance in life to ride a motorcycle. My life was safe, perfect, and boring with Steve."

Rachel called Eli. Darnell heard snatches of the conversation as Elizabeth loudly tried to talk Rachel out of it. He heard 'professional boundaries' and he heard Eli call motorcycles organ donor machines.

Rachel concluded the phone call, saying, "I appreciate all your advice, but it's my life to make my own mistakes. I'll see you this evening. Tell Buckeye I'll pet him when I get home." Rachel hung up the phone. "Oy Vey! She thinks she's my mother."

Chapter 38

As Darnell dug his extra helmet and his leather jacket out of the closet, Rachel cleaned up the supplies from the infusion, placed them in an infectious waste bag, and packed up her nurse's bag with butterflies in her stomach.

They rode the elevator down together.

Rachel touched Darnell on his shoulder. "I remember riding this elevator with you last spring. You could hardly stand up. I was terrified that you were going to pass out."

"I didn't realize that I was that sick. I have this tough macho image of my body being able to withstand anything, even losing half my blood. It took me over a month before I felt well enough to do anything. I'm learning how precious and fragile life is."

"You may be learning your body's vulnerabilities; I'm learning the human body's resilience. I am always amazed at what a human body can endure and still survive. I've seen so many patients knocking at death's door bounce back. I don't know if it is the body itself, or the spirit or life force within a person that keeps them going."

"It may have something to do with God. God healed me when I was knocking at death's door." He headed towards his motorcycle.

Rachel headed to her car to stow her nursing supplies, jacket, and lab coat in the trunk. Her body trembled. *What the hell am I doing? I'm becoming a motorcycle mama. I've always told Shelly everything. I can't tell her about this, at least for ten years or so.*

"Rachel, I'd like you to meet Rusty. She's not as rusty as she was when I first got her. I may have to change her name next year." He helped Rachel put his leather jacket on. "The wind can bite once we start going fast."

She exclaimed, "Fast? You promised not to go fast! Remember, this is my first time ever on a motorcycle."

"I'll take care of you." Darnell helped her put the green helmet on. "It matches your green eyes." He leaned his face close to hers to adjust the straps, close enough that she could feel his breath on her face.

"This is the most important part, making sure the helmet fits snugly." A stray curl slipped out of her helmet, and he very gently put it back.

Again, she felt that familiar tingling down to her groin.

"After I get on, you sit behind me. Put your feet on those foot pegs and keep them there. Be careful not to touch this metal exhaust pipe, it can get ridiculously hot and burn right through your pants. Once you're seated, put your arms around my hips or waist and hold tight. That's my favorite part." He grinned. "Don't be afraid of the turns. Just lean into them with me. You won't fall."

Rachel hopped onto the seat and put her arms around Darnell's waist. The insides of her thighs hugged the outsides of Darnell's thighs. The engine started with a loud, throaty growl. Rachel felt the vibration of the cycle and the thrumpy exhaust sounds in her legs, abdomen, and chest. The bike rattled a bit as Darnell slowly weaved his way out of the parking lot and onto Lakeshore Blvd. The traffic was light, and Rachel watched Darnell's hands and feet, marveling at the work involved in driving a motorcycle. His left hand and foot changed the gears, and his right hand and foot manned the brakes. His entire body commandeered the cycle. Her body relaxed into the exhilaration of the open road, with her senses ripening into focus. She felt the warm breeze caressing her cheeks as she smelled exhaust fumes from Rusty and the other cars on the road and inhaled the delicious aromas wafting from the Italian food and burger joints along the road. She noticed the blueness of the sky with the orange, red, purple, and yellow trees flying past. She loved the feel of her arms around Darnell's taut waist. She felt utterly safe and totally vulnerable, completely alive, and acutely aware of her own mortality.

He started to increase his speed when they got to the two-lane highway leading into North Chagrin Reservation. When they rounded the curves, the cycle slanted as Darnell had warned her. At first, she tried to fight the curves by leaning out of them but learned to enjoy the curves by squeezing Darnell's waist a little tighter and putting her helmeted head close to his shoulders. Eventually they arrived at the ancient woods. He stopped the cycle and helped her off.

Rachel pulled off her helmet. "I think I'm in love."

Darnell took her hands. "I've been in love with you since the day I saw you walk into the dialysis unit."

Rachel stammered. "I meant I love riding your motorcycle." *Is that really the truth? I think I'm falling for him. How could it possibly work? Am I leading him on?*

He took her in his arms and hugged her anyway. "Let's go watch the leaves. First, take my jacket off. It is too warm for walking in the woods today."

They walked along a path carpeted with multicolored leaves and moving shadows created by the tree branches swaying in the sunlight. The yellow, orange, and red trees on each side of the path provided a sheltering arbor. The leaves crunching under their feet released the pungent, sweet aroma of autumn. Darnell stopped and took a deep breath. "I'm glad to be alive to see another autumn." After walking for twenty minutes or so, they arrived at a picnic table underneath a canopy of trees.

Darnell climbed on top of the picnic table, lay on his back, and patted the area next to him. "Come and see."

She climbed on top of the picnic table and lay next to him, cupping her hands behind her head. She gazed at the treetops reaching to forever, their branches piercing the sky. The myriads of leaves floating to the earth, floating, glinting, and shining in the sunlight, mesmerized her. Scattered leaves exploded with color as the sunlight caught them, turning them into tiny floating lanterns. Other leaves shimmered like gold coins drifting to earth. She took deep breaths, trying to gather the experience inside. "Wow."

Rachel looked at him. "Thanks for bringing me." She pointed to the treetops. "Look at those branches hugging each other. They're all connected."

Darnell turned towards her. "I bet if you could see their roots tangled together under the ground, you'd really see their connections. I read somewhere that trees communicate with each other. Native American mothers would teach their children that if they got lost in the forest to just hold on to the closest tree and the mother would touch the tree closest to her, and the trees would lead her to her child."

Rachel chortled. "Smart mothers. Kept the children from wandering away too far and really getting lost. I like the idea of trees communicating though. I wonder if they tell each other stories of the human lives that have lived and died under their watch over the centuries. Do they laugh and remind each other of particularly crazy humans that have trampled their roots?"

Darnell shrugged. "Trees may find stories of the squirrels, birds, bugs, and fungi more interesting than human dramas. In fact, I think the reason why these trees are still around is because there weren't too many humans trampling their roots. If I were a tree, I'd be afraid of humans. We're the ones with the chainsaws."

As they lay there several leaves landed on their bodies.

Rachel felt a faint flutter and placed her hand over her abdomen. Darnell noticed and asked if she felt the baby move.

She shook her head. "I think it was just a falling leaf."

"When my sister was pregnant, she told me the first time she felt the twins it felt like a feather, faint and almost imperceptible."

Rachel put her hand over her womb for a few moments and shook her head. "I think it really was just a leaf." She pictured the fetus swimming and flipping like she had seen in the last ultrasound. She thought about the life she was carrying and thought of all the lives the trees had witnessed and was filled with awe at the mystery and privilege of being part of the overflowing big life around her.

The two of them lay on the picnic table, still and quiet. They didn't disturb the leaves that continued landing on their bodies. Eventually, clouds moved in, and the sun shifted to the horizon, lending a chill to the air.

Rachel started to shiver. "I'm getting cold. We better head back."

As they walked back to Rusty, Darnell put his arm around her shoulder to warm her. "I should have brought the leather jacket with us. I always forget how cool it gets in autumn once the sun starts setting."

As they walked along the path, Darnell told Rachel that he loved to come to the woods at any season. "They teach me how to live in the different seasons of my life. Watching the leaves leap from the trees with abandon teaches me to let go of all the things I cling to. Winter woods teach me to stand naked as I wait for spring to come."

Rachel nodded. "I think your time on dialysis is one of your life's winters. A transplant will arrive. Spring will come." They walked quietly.

Rachel picked up a perfectly colored leaf with reds, yellows, and greens. "In my whole life, I've never taken the time to watch the leaves fall. I've always been too busy, too driven to accomplish something…not sure exactly what I thought was so important. This afternoon reminds me of another afternoon when I was a child, home alone with my father. He was already sick, not working anymore. It was a warm spring afternoon, and he invited me to the front yard to lie on the grass with him under the trees and watch the leaves budding on the branches. We lay under those trees all afternoon. I'll always remember that afternoon. Maybe this one too."

"Did you see any buds bursting forth?"

"Nah, they were just there. You'd think we'd be able to see it. Leaves burst from buds overnight in spring. We watched a bird build her nest though.

The sun set as they rode back. Rachel watched the multi-colored sunset sky fade into blinking city lights whizzing by.

Rachel thanked Darnell, returned his leather jacket and helmet, and gave him a quick hug. "Thank you."

Darnell smiled. "Let's do it again."

As Rachel turned to leave at the lighted entrance of the apartment building, Shanita and the boys arrived. He picked his nephews up and hugged them. The twins remembered Rachel and smiled and waved at her from their perches in Darnell's arms.

When Darnell introduced Rachel as his infusion nurse, Shanita tilted her head, squinted, and looked at Darnell. "I didn't know you could get IVs on motorcycles."

Rachel explained, "I gave him the IV in his apartment and then Darnell took me for a ride. I see you are wearing scrubs. Do you work in healthcare?"

"I'm working as a nurses' aide but hoping to be a nurse one day."

Rachel smiled. "Would you be interested in learning how to give Darnell his antibiotics? You'd have to learn how to put an IV in Darnell's arm. Do you think you could do that?"

Darnell frowned.

Shanita smiled the same familiar smile that often radiated from Darnell's face. "I would love to. Can you teach me in the evening?"

"We can work that out. Darnell needs his next infusion the day after tomorrow." She handed her card to Shanita. "Call this number tomorrow and the secretary will find a convenient time for me to teach you. It may take more than one lesson. Darnell will need infusions four days a week for the next four weeks."

Shanita looked at her brother. "We see him nearly every day anyway."

Darnell walked Rachel to her car.

Rachel touched his arm. "Don't be disappointed with Shanita giving your infusions. It's a lucky chance for me to get to know your sister. I'd rather spend time with you off the clock anyway, and for sure I'd like another motorcycle ride."

Darnell gently took her head into his hands and kissed her forehead. That kiss burned her forehead the entire drive back to Elizabeth's.

- Chapter 39 -

Two nights later, Rachel showed up at Darnell's apartment to give Shanita her first infusion lesson. Shanita hadn't arrived yet because Rachel appeared forty-five minutes earlier than the scheduled appointment time. (It wasn't like Rachel to be early for anything.) Darnell was studying but quickly closed his textbook. The aroma of cooked onions and garlic and the music of The Marriage of Figaro playing in the background greeted Rachel.

"Mmm…what smells so good?

"Pork casserole for Shanita and her boys. She's coming straight here from work, so she won't have time to cook. I hid the garlic and onions in the casserole with lots of vegetables. Lester and Clarence will eat anything if there are noodles mixed in and they're hungry enough. Would you like some?"

Rachel's stomach grumbled and the casserole smelled delicious. "No thanks, I don't eat pork." She walked to his kitchen table, put down a clean pad, and started setting up her supplies. "So nice of you to cook for them. I don't know much about toddlers, but I'd be surprised to see them eat garlic, onions, and vegetables in the same dish."

"I confess I made the casserole for you, but it never occurred to me you might not eat pork."

Rachel tried to explain. "I don't keep Kosher per se, but avoiding pork might be a Jewish genetic predisposition. In Asia, they eat dogs. I know that idea would turn your stomach. That's what pork's like for me. I like your choice of music. The Marriage of Figaro is one of my favorites."

Darnel smiled. "I'm learning that once you hear a piece of

music a few times, it carves a channel inside, and you don't just hear it, but experience it as it travels inside. I'm starting to enjoy opera, but the stories are silly. Shanita won't be here for a half hour. Come sit with me on the balcony and tell me about your day."

They sat on the folding chairs and watched the Great Lake. A large barge lumbered in the distance; a few sailboats glided closer to shore. Seagulls screeched overhead.

Darnell leaned back on his chair, hands behind his head, legs stretched out, eager for a good story. "Any new dialysis gossip or drama? Any scolding or new rules from Ms. Leggett? Did Buckeye bite any patients, get tangled in dialysis lines, or poop on the floor?"

Rachel sighed. "I sent a patient to the ER because he was having chest pain. The ER doc sent him right back stating that he was fine and just needed dialysis. The patient returned by cab, but he still didn't look right." She shook her head. "I knew something was wrong, but I didn't know what else to do, so we got a new setup and started him back on dialysis. When ER doctors send patients back to a dialysis unit, they don't realize that outpatient dialysis units run on very tight schedules. Putting this patient back on the machine threw the entire afternoon schedule off. It was a mess. Pandemonium. No one wants to have their chair changed or get on the machine late, or worse, get off the machine later than their off time. The worst part of the story though, is that the patient arrested thirty minutes after restarting dialysis. We did CPR and called the ambulance again. The EMTs shook their heads when they realized they were picking up the same patient they had dropped off in the ER two hours previously."

"Do you think he'll live?"

"I think so. When the ambulance arrived, he was awake and complaining of worse chest pain. I think we broke one of his ribs with the CPR. I don't know why the ER doc didn't keep him the first time around. It takes twenty-four hours for a basic workup for chest pain. Ms. Leggett came out and yelled at me for sending two patients to the hospital because hospitalizations look bad on her monthly quality control reports."

Darnell laughed. "She always emerges from her den to yell after the ambulance arrives. What did you tell her?"

"I told her that it was just one patient twice, and that hospitalizations look better on the monthly quality reports than deaths. I wish I had the balls not to accept the patient back to the dialysis unit from the ER. In my gut I knew something was wrong. Eli always tells me to trust my gut, but Ms. Leggett wouldn't have backed me up. She thinks the doctor is always right. I know if Eli or Dr. Burnouf were in the unit today, they wouldn't have accepted the patient back. I probably shouldn't be telling you all the politics and ins and outs of the day-to-day in the dialysis unit."

"No worries. You aren't telling me anything I don't know. I see everything from the vantage point of my dialysis chair. Maybe someday you'll have Ms. Leggett's job and will be calling the shots. Or maybe you'll become a nurse practitioner like Eli."

Rachel pulled out her phone. "The big news today though, is that I put a deposit on a tiny house in Cleveland Hts. It's behind one of those old mansions. It was a carriage house or maid's quarters a hundred years ago. It has two bedrooms, and the kitchen was remodeled with a washer and dryer in it. It overlooks a creek. Perfect house to bring a newborn to. I'm excited to be moving out on my own. I moved in with Steve right after college, so I've never had the experience of living on my own in my own house. Here's a picture of it." She handed her phone to Darnell. "Look at all those big old trees around it. My move-in date is November first.

Darnell looked at the picture. "It looks nice. It needs a motorcycle in the garage though."

Rachel narrowed her eyes. "If you think you are moving in with me because you took me on an amazing motorcycle ride, think again."

"I wasn't thinking of moving *myself* in with you, just my motorcycle. Today I stopped by Howard's Cash Flash Pawn shop to negotiate the pawning of Rusty to bail out my brother. I discovered that the situation isn't as simple as I thought. My brother's bail is ten thousand dollars because he already has a felony. I hoped Howard would give me that amount because I think Rusty is worth twenty thousand or more. He told me he is trying to run a business and that the most he'll give me is five thousand." He shrugged his shoulders. "No special breaks for a fellow dialysis patient. Even with the five thousand, I still have to pay a bail bondsman five hundred dollars for the remaining five thousand dollars needed. The worst part though is Howard plans to charge me one hundred dollars a month to store Rusty. I can't afford that."

"Sounds like bailing out your brother is going to be a major hassle."

"I'm doing it for Mama. If it were up to me, I'd let Will sit in jail. Some of his friends are dangerous, and he makes poor choices. His stint in prison didn't teach him to make better choices. Even though the Cuyahoga County jail isn't the safest place to be, I'm convinced that he is safer in jail than out on the streets. So, can I store Rusty in your garage? I won't be able to drive her. I'm required to leave the title, registration, and keys with Howard until the bail is returned with my brother's court appearance. I might visit Rusty at your house occasionally…maybe every day, just to make sure she is okay."

"I didn't even look at the garage when I signed the lease. I'll check it out tomorrow and let you know. Hoping there will be space for my car *and* Rusty. In the lease I agreed to mow the lawn and keep the yard looking nice. I've never done yard work before. Would you be willing to do yard work in exchange for sheltering Rusty?"

"I've been doing Mama's yard work since I was eight years old. No problem. Even though my haggling with Howard didn't turn out as I hoped, he offered me a job in his shop. Tamika's son was working for him, but he went away to college. Howard and I will need to switch our dialysis schedules so I can cover the shop when he is on the machine and vice versa. It will be refreshing to finally work for someone who knows what it's like to be a dialysis patient."

"I bet working at the Cash Flash will be interesting. Howard always has some unusual stories to tell."

"Interesting, maybe. I'm just glad to have a job again."

Shanita arrived with Clarence and Lester. The two boys ran and jumped into Darnell's arms. He served the casserole in bowls to his nephews.

They looked at the mixture with the vegetables, wrinkled their noses, squealed "Eeeew," jumped off their chairs, and ran to their little toy chest.

Rachel laughed. "I guess you didn't fool them by hiding the vegetables and onions with the noodles."

Darnell made grilled cheese sandwiches and cut up apples for his nephews. He fed them as they played on the floor with their trucks and cars. As Darnell took care of his nephews, Rachel taught Shanita how to give the infusion to her brother. She had written up a step-by-step instruction sheet specifically for Shanita. Rachel obsessed about anything and everything that could possibly go wrong, realizing that she preferred to do things herself, realizing that she had become a control freak. Shanita listened intently, asking many questions. As Rachel walked her through the instruction sheet, she noticed Shanita's hands trembling.

"Am I making you nervous?"

"I'm afraid of making a mistake. Next to the twins, I love Darnell like my own life. What if I make a mistake? What if I hurt him?"

Rachel nodded. "You'll do fine. I'll be here each time until you are comfortable and safe doing it on your own."

Finally, it was time for Shanita to insert the butterfly needle into Darnell's arm. They called Darnell to the table. Clarence and Lester's heads popped up and they followed Darnell to the table to watch their mom put a needle in their uncle's arm. They were intent and quiet as their eyes peered over the top of the table. Clarence put his hand on his uncle's thigh for reassurance; just like his mother did when he had to get a shot. Darnell started making faces and pretending to cry for his nephews' benefit. His nephews snickered.

Darnell instructed Shanita, "First you put the tourniquet on, not too tight but tight enough for my veins to start popping up."

Shanita shook her head. "I don't be needing two teachers now." She washed her hands, put on some gloves, put on the tourniquet, and looked for a good vein.

Rachel guided Shanita step by step in inserting the needle, taping it in place and hooking it up to the bag of antibiotic solution.

When the IV was infusing, Shanita sat back and smiled. "I can't believe I just did that. You're the best teacher."

"You're the best student ever." This was the first time Rachel had ever taught anyone to do anything medical, and she found it quite satisfying.

Clarence and Lester returned to playing with their cars and Rachel, Darnell, and Shanita sat at the table as the antibiotic infused. Rachel watched the twins playing with their cars. "Do you have any advice for a single mom-to-be? I don't know how you do it with twins."

"I couldn't have done it without Darnell. Their baby daddy wanted nothing to do with them nor me, however the courts are making him pay child support, which is a good thing, because the twins are getting more expensive to raise with each passing month."

"Did you nurse them when they were infants?"

"I knew it was healthier and cheaper to nurse them. The worst part is that I didn't get a minute of sleep the first year of their lives. Things are easier now because they taught themselves to sleep at night and they play well together."

"What's the hardest part?"

"I'm not at the point where I can answer that question. I'm still learning as I go along. Everyone tells me that when they're little, the problems are little. Right now, the hardest part is keeping them safe and amused. The days are long and boring. Sometimes a day lasts a thousand years. Even so, they are my life. I love them." Rachel liked Shanita and hoped someday they would become friends.

- Chapter 40 -

November arrived and it was time to pawn Rusty. Darnell took Rachel on one final ride to Chagrin Falls. It was a chilly, gray, damp early November day, and they shivered. They bought themselves hot coffee and walked down the steps to the Falls viewing area. Water from the falls splashed them, chilling them even further. Rachel told Darnell that perhaps his leather jacket was warm in October, but today she needed a snowsuit. Darnell told her that today was the perfect day to ease the pain of pawning Rusty.

"You got that right. Not sure if I'll ever get warm again, not sure I ever want to ride Rusty again."

"Come spring and the first sunny warm day you'll jump at the chance," Darnell assured her.

A few days later, Darnell brought his motorcycle registration, title, keys, and license to Harold and collected $5,000, one-half of the bail money. He expected the process of bailing out his brother to take one to two hours but not an entire day. He first had to deal with the bail bondsman for the remaining $5000, who gave him the once-over. The bondsman checked his income, which was just social security disability and a few paystubs from the Cash Flash Pawn shop. He wasn't impressed with the picture Darnell showed him of Rusty. He wanted a copy of his lease and utility bills.

Darnell went home and returned with the paperwork. Luckily his credit rating was good, and he had never gotten into trouble with the law. Darnell signed piles of papers with microscopic printing. He tried to read them but didn't fully understand them. He wondered how anyone could, and wondered how such legalese could be legal. He had never borrowed so much money in his life and hated the thought of being in debt. Darnell forked over the last five hundred dollars in his savings account, fearing that he'd never see that money again. He just hoped he'd have Rusty again come spring.

If Will doesn't show for his court date, I'll owe the full five thousand and lose Rusty. His stomach churned.

Finally, at the end of the day the guards escorted Will out in civilian clothes that were three sizes too big. Darnell laughed when he saw his brother dwarfed by the large men's clothes. The brothers hugged. Darnell was genuinely glad to see Will and felt a slight pang of guilt for holding on to Rusty the past few months. He realized how much he loved his brother.

Will didn't hold a grudge and was delighted just to be free. He was full of smiles. "Thank you, bro. Glad to bust out of that crowbar hotel."

"How bad was it? Mama was convinced you would die in there, has been praying up a storm, and has all her homies praying. I think I was the weak link in the answer to her prayers. I didn't want to pawn Rusty until all the leaves had fallen. How bad was it? Did any of the corrections officers abuse you?"

"Nah, things were cool. I played lots of cards and made some new connections. The officers were on their best behavior after the reports of eight deaths in the jail last year."

"I'm not happy to hear of new connections. What do you mean by that?"

"Nothing…just new friends."

"What do you think will happen when you go to court?"

"My lawyer keeps saying I'll get a reduced sentence if I tell the court the names of the suppliers in the neighborhood. Can I stay with you? I lost my lease when I was in jail, and all my belongings were stolen."

"I love you Will, but I don't think I could take the stress of keeping tabs on you. I'm dropping you off at Mama's."

"Aw shit. Mama be dragging me to church."

"It might do you good. When I was in ICU, Jesus sat next to me on a park bench. Mama might have some better connections than the ones in jail."

"Let's go out for a beer before you drop me off."

"First, I'll bring you to my apartment so I can give you some clothes that fit."

They revisited the last time they saw each other when the police came.

Will got very serious. "I'm sorry it happened. I thought about you all the time in jail. If I knew my coming to your apartment that day would cause you to be beaten up, I would never have come. I thought you were angry with me when you didn't come to visit me."

"I'll admit, I was angry. That beating cracked my skull and ruined my fistula. I didn't feel like seeing you for a while. Did Mama tell you about my hospitalizations?"

Will nodded. "Did you get my letter telling you how sorry I was? I was hoping you'd come see me after that. I wanted to apologize in person."

"I forgave you after I received the letter. I'm incarcerated on a dialysis machine three days a week. Any free time I have is spent taking care of the twins or seeing Rachel. If you are truly sorry, stay clean and show up for your court appearance so I don't end up in the poor house."

Afterwards, Darnell and Will went out for a beer or two, and lost count. They laughed and joked like they used to when they were younger. Will beat Darnell in several games of pool. Darnell updated Will about Mama and J.R.'s marriage, about Rachel and the potential for love, and Shanita and the twins. Darnell hadn't talked so much non-stop in a long time. He talked of his college courses and how much he loved learning again. It was long past last call at the bar when Darnell and

Will headed to Mama's. Mama hugged Will with tears in her eyes and introduced Will to J.R. Will would be sleeping in his old bedroom until his court date. Mama then gave Darnell one of her trademark hugs that lasted forever, thanking him for the sacrifices he made to bail Will out of jail.

- Chapter 41 -

Rachel had moved out of Elizabeth's home into the tiny house under the big trees a few weeks previously, and Elizabeth missed her company. Her house seemed colder, lonelier, and emptier than it felt before the evening Rachel showed up at her front door soaking wet. She was glad at least to have Buckeye keeping her company. Today she had a follow-up appointment with Dr. Max Burnouf. This appointment was a major source of anxiety for her. First there had been the argument when he suspected she tried to commit suicide with her low blood sugar reaction. And then there was his HIPAA-violating conversation with her daughter Becky about her healthcare choices. What made her the most nervous though, were her recent labs showing that her kidney function continued its steady decline. Elizabeth dreaded this appointment so much that she rescheduled it three times and spent a few weeks considering switching to a different nephrologist in town. She made appointments with two of them and then canceled them when she realized that even though things had gone south between her and Max, she trusted him. Who else could she go to? He was her friend. She was nervous about confronting him and seeing him face to face. Was he still angry with her?

Today she took the elevator. Her fatigue was getting worse. Buckeye accompanied her. As they walked down the hall toward his office, she instructed him, "Now, when that bald man with the glasses walks into the room, you need to make a low growl. I know that is not in your nature, but it's important you do that today."

Buckeye nodded his head in understanding as he walked next to Elizabeth. Buckeye enjoyed the attention he received from the secretary, medical assistants, and nurse. The nurse ushered them into the exam room. Elizabeth declined to sit on the exam table or put on a hospital gown. She wanted to be on equal footing when confronting Max. Buckeye sat quietly next to her.

She didn't have to wait long. Max noticed Buckeye and went to pet him. "Glad to finally meet you Buckeye. I hope you are taking good care of Eli." He looked at Elizabeth. "All the patients in the dialysis unit talk about Buckeye. I can see why he is so popular. He's quite charming."

"He's a bad dog today, not behaving as instructed."

"What was he supposed to do?"

"He was supposed to growl when he saw your face. I'm going to have to train him better."

Max tilted his head. "Growl when he saw me? Are you angry because I told Becky that you were planning to avoid dialysis?"

"It not only hurt that you went behind my back, but you broke the law."

He looked into her eyes and spoke with such tenderness that Elizabeth's eyes filled with tears. "I told Becky because I care about you. Sometimes a person needs to break a law to do the right thing. I knew your daughters would talk some sense into you. I suspected you were angry with me when you canceled the past three appointments. And you've become an escape artist in dodging me in the dialysis units. I miss rounding with you."

Elizabeth smiled. "Dodging you was easy. Your secretary has been sending me your schedule for years."

Max asked her about her symptoms; her appetite, how she was sleeping, and how she was feeling overall. She reported that her appetite continued to be great. The thing that bothered her most was the fatigue. She told him she wasn't sure how long she could continue working.

He noted that her blood count had continued to drop, and it was time to start her on Aranesp, a medication to stimulate her bone marrow to make more blood cells. "That might help your fatigue for a time, but you know as well as I do that patients often start dialysis because of the fatigue." He listened to her heart and lungs and was pleased that she wasn't retaining any fluid.

He asked to examine her fistula. "I saw the report from the surgeon a few weeks back." Elizabeth held out her arm. "The fistula started out looking like it would develop well for dialysis with a good thrill and bruit, but it just shut down one afternoon for no reason. I returned to the surgeon a few days ago and his new plan is to put a graft in right before I need to start dialysis. He said he'd send you the report."

He gently took her arm into his hands and palpated the now defunct fistula. "I'm sorry it didn't work."

"Max, I saw my labs last week. It's terrible knowing everything that I know. I wish I were a bit more naïve."

"Working in health care is a double-edged sword. We know all about the diseases, but that doesn't protect our bodies from taking the same trajectory as many of our patients. The body's inevitable deterioration is difficult to accept."

After a long moment, Max shifted uncomfortably in his chair. "I have a confession to make."

She looked at him expectantly, intrigued.

He took a deep breath. "I couldn't sleep last night; I was nervous about your visit today. I know I overreacted to your low blood sugar reaction. I was afraid to lose you. You are more than just a patient to me, more than just a friend. We have worked together for years; our children grew up together, and now we're both alone and go home every evening to an empty house. Will you come out to dinner with me?"

Elizabeth was flabbergasted. This was not what she expected.

She tilted her head. "Are you asking me out on a date?"

"I guess…I feel like a teenager. I haven't asked a woman out since I asked my wife to the prom when I was seventeen."

"I need to make a consultation." She looked at Buckeye. "What do you think? Do you think it's a good idea for me to go on a date with my doctor, my boss, and particularly good friend?" Buckeye barked and Elizabeth chuckled, "I didn't train him to do that. In fact, he is trained to bark only when my blood sugars are too high or too low, or I'm in trouble in some way."

"Shall we check your blood sugar?"

"No, my blood sugar has been in range lately. Maybe Buckeye barked because he sensed my anxiety."

Max looked at Buckeye and petted him. "Tell Eli that she'll be safe with me."

Buckeye barked again.

Elizabeth took a deep breath. "I didn't date at all when my girls were teenagers because I didn't want to complicate their lives. Now that they're grown, I'm afraid to date because I don't want to saddle anyone with my health issues. I don't want to be a burden to anyone, nor have the shame of a partner watching my inevitable decline."

Max shook his head. "We're both aging and declining predictably. It's part of the cycle of life. I'm no spring chicken either. I have radioactive seeds in my prostate, high blood pressure, and arthritis all over my body. We'll hold each other up as we deteriorate in unison."

"Have you dated since your wife died?"

"No. Just working up the courage to ask you out gave me insomnia. I'm not interested in dating just any pretty face. I can't imagine starting from scratch at my age with a stranger, but I know you. We have a history, an understanding, and we laugh at the same things."

"That's true, but what about all the arguments we had over

the years? What if we argue every time we see each other?"

"I don't remember the arguments; I remember the laughs."

"I'll go out to eat with you under one condition. You are not allowed to monitor the food I order or judge what I eat. You can't be my nephrologist, just be my friend."

"Point well taken. If you agree to date me, I'm going to ask you to switch your care to my partner. I've already demonstrated to you that I've lost any objectivity with regards to you, even to the point of breaking the law. I'd rather be your friend than your nephrologist."

Elizabeth whispered. "I'd rather have you as my friend too. I've missed you."

"It's a deal. Are you free this Friday evening?"

"I'm free every Friday evening."

"I'll pick you up at six. Will that give you enough time?"

"It depends on when I finish work. I usually walk Buckeye for an hour when I get home."

"Call me when you get home from work, and we'll walk Buckeye together."

Elizabeth squinted her eyes. "Aren't your days longer than mine?"

"I've cut back on my schedule. I don't have the strength and stamina that I used to. I'm thinking of retiring."

"It's usually dark when I walk Buckeye these days. Are your eyes okay? How is your balance? I'd hate to have you end up in the hospital on our first date."

"Stop it, Eli! We'll have to hold each other up. I know all about your neuropathy and retinopathy. *You* shouldn't be out walking a dog alone in the dark these days. Now that I think of it, I might have to walk Buckeye with you every evening."

"I also walk him in the dark every morning."

"Oh, dear, that means I might have to move in to help you walk Buckeye mornings and evenings."

"Don't rush things Max. Now you're scaring me. See you Friday."

Elizabeth walked out of the office wondering if she'd be able to sleep between now and Friday.

- Chapter 42 --

Rachel's cottage was in a quiet parklike setting with woods and a gully in the back. It was partially furnished. She found an ancient wooden table in the kitchen and a comfortable couch in the living room. She loved sitting on the couch and gazing out the front window at the trees in the yard. There was enough room in her garage for her car *and* Darnell's motorcycle. He came often to visit Rusty. Well, that's what they both pretended. They loved spending time together. Rachel looked forward to his visits and often had a million things to tell him the minute he arrived.

The nesting instinct kicked in. Uncertain of the sex of her baby, she painted the nursery a pale green because she had read that green is soothing to babies. She started shopping for baby furniture, baby toys, and imagined her life as a mother. She frequented the public library down the street, carrying home piles of books for the expectant mother. She devoured pregnancy and parenting books while her nursing journals gathered dust in a pile in the corner. She thrilled at the pictures of the developing fetus each week of her pregnancy.

The morning nausea subsided, and Rachel felt good. She was five months along. During Rachel's last ultrasound, Dr. O'Keefe told her that she was carrying a boy. She felt her son flipping and moving all the time, so alive and active. Dr. O'Keefe reassured her at her visits that everything was progressing normally.

Rachel often put her hand over her abdomen to feel her son's little kicks and nudges. One day, when Darnell was visiting, she told him, "That day in the woods, when I thought it was just a leaf falling, was really the first time I felt the baby move. You knew before I did. Someday I'll tell him that initially I thought he was just a leaf. I've named him Leif for now."

The friendship between Rachel and Darnell blossomed as winter set in. Rachel's cottage had a fireplace, and Darnell would gather wood in the woods behind the cottage whenever he visited. They would sit in front of the fire talking, sometimes kissing, and cuddling. It dawned on Rachel that her relationship with Darnell wasn't *just* a friendship. She found herself desiring him and felt a delicious churning in her abdomen when he was around.

The festival of Hanukkah arrived, and Darnell came over every evening to light the Hanukkah candles. He read about the Maccabees and the miracle of the oil. He learned the prayers for lighting the candles in English and Rachel would recite them in Hebrew. Rachel loved that he was genuinely interested in the holiday, and she enjoyed the quiet evenings with him basking in the glow of the Hanukkah candles.

On the eighth night of Hanukkah, the warm fire crackling in the fireplace and the eight candles on the menorah added a romantic golden glow to the evening. Darnell pulled out a dreidel that he purchased at a Judaica store and asked Rachel to teach him how to play.

Rachel taught him how to spin the Dreidel and explained that it was sort of like playing dice or craps, except instead of numbers, there were Hebrew letters on each side of the dreidel top. She told him that the Hebrew letters on the dreidel make an acronym in Hebrew, meaning "A great miracle happened there." The game starts out with everyone putting a token into the pot. People take turns spinning the dreidel and whatever letter is up when the top stops spinning tells the person what to do. If it lands on the letter *Nun*, the person does nothing. If it lands on the letter *Shin*, the person puts a token in the pot. If it lands on the letter *Hay*, the person takes half of the pot. If it lands on the letter *Gimel*, the person takes everything in the pot. Rachel explained that usually they played this with pennies or Hanukkah gelt, which are foil-covered chocolate coins. "We can't play with Hanukkah gelt because you can't eat chocolate. How about pennies?"

"Pennies are boring. Let's wager our clothes. That would make this game exciting. If the Dreidel lands on *Gimel*, I take all your clothes off, if it lands on *Hay*, I just take half of your clothes off. If it lands on *Shin*, I put one of your clothes back on. If it lands on *Nun*, I do nothing and try to spin better next time."

Rachel laughed. "I know this game has been played with varying rules and tokens over the centuries, but you may be the first person in history who thought of using clothes as the stakes. Wagering our clothes guarantees that we'll both be naked in a few spins."

Darnell rubbed his hands together. "What a great game, let's get started."

Rachel felt hot and moist at the thought of Darnell carefully removing her clothes and having sex with him. She had fantasized about having sex with Darnell for the past few months, surprised at her increased sexual interest even while pregnant.

"I'm scared. This game would change everything. We would no longer just be friends. I would also be breaking some professional boundaries."

"Rachel, you broke that boundary long ago, perhaps that first day you drove me home from dialysis. We'll always be friends, but after tonight, we'll be friends *and* lovers. Just being your friend isn't working for me anyway. Don't be afraid. I promise to take good care of you." He leaned over and kissed her.

She melted. She wanted to resist but couldn't find a single

pocket of resistance within her. She wanted him.

Rachel watched as Darnell prepared the playing area for the Dreidel game. He took the blanket from the couch and laid it on the carpet in front of the fireplace. He placed cushions around and then put the Dreidel in between them. She sensed his excitement in the preparations. Darnell spun the dreidel first, and it landed on Gimel. "A lucky spin!"

That was the end of the dreidel game. Darnell took Rachel's palms in his hands and, with his thumbs, massaged her palms slowly. She found herself getting even more aroused at that simple act. The skin on her entire body came alive. He carefully removed her sweater, and then her bra. He kissed her breasts, murmuring how beautiful they were. He kissed her neck and nibbled on her ears. He took off her socks and massaged her feet like he did her palms, kissing each toe. He then gently slid off her jeans and underwear. He sat back on his knees in the mellow candlelight and admired her body with his hands, paying special attention to Rachel's baby bump. He put his hands over her womb for a while until he felt the baby move. "Little Leif, I haven't met you yet, but I promise to take care of you too." He then massaged Rachel's thighs and in between her legs.

Rachel arched her back and moaned. She sat up. "I need to get your clothes off."

She imitated how he had removed her clothes by massaging his palms first, and then she removed his sweatshirt. She kissed and sucked his breasts and moved her hand down his abdomen and into his pants, admiring his erect shaft. She massaged it as she removed his pants and underwear. She didn't get to the point of removing his socks and massaging his feet because he was already too excited. He took over and had her lie down again.

With renewed vigor he resumed massaging Rachel with special emphasis on her thighs and groin until she moaned in orgasm, ripples and waves rolling through her body. "I love you, Rachel."

He looked into her eyes, and she lost herself in his gaze. "I love you too Darnell." She kissed him and pulled him to her.

He moved inside of her in a slow rhythm until they both orgasmed simultaneously.

He lay on top of her, spent. "Rachel, Rachel, Rachel."

They lay entwined in front of the fireplace for a long time. The Hanukkah candles burnt out and the embers in the fireplace grew cold.

Darnell sat up and looked tenderly into Rachel's eyes. "That dreidel really is a game of miracles. A great miracle happened here tonight."

Rachel invited him to spend the night. "I need to get up at 3:30 am tomorrow to get to work. I hope that doesn't disturb your sleep."

He rubbed his chin. "Hmm, I'll have to think about that one long and hard," as he headed to her bedroom and jumped on her bed.

Together they burrowed under a pile of covers, hugging each other's naked bodies. She told him this was the best Hanukkah she ever celebrated as she snuggled into him. Rachel fell asleep with the sound of Darnell's fistula whispering in her ear like a waterfall with each beat of his heart.

When Rachel rose early the following morning, she noticed pink spotting on her underwear as she got ready for work. She looked up her new symptom in the pile of maternity books on her kitchen table and was reassured that a little spotting was a normal occurrence in pregnancy. She kissed Darnell on his forehead and whispered, "I'll see you later today at your favorite place."

The roads would be slippery and slow. She put on a pad for the spotting and threw a few extra in her purse, just in case. She set off early. It was dark, the roads were slick, and visibility was poor. Even though the windshield wipers worked noisily and furiously, she could only see a few feet ahead of her car in the dark. Her car crept along the vanishing road. She passed the time remembering and replaying the previous evening. She recalled the moments of him massaging her palm and gently removing her clothes. She got hot and moist remembering their lovemaking. She tried to pinpoint the moment she started falling in love with him. *I think it was the day he waited outside the dialysis unit, worried about me, after Ethel died. No, it was before that. There was always this solid, quiet presence about him that attracted me to him. I always wanted to be near him.*

She arrived at work and discovered that everything was delayed because of the blizzard. No one had arrived on time. As she started rounding on her patients, she felt some back and abdominal cramping. This cramping was worse than any menstrual cramps. *The spotting might be normal, but this cramping is not. Shit, I'm miscarrying.*

She finished the first shift of patients, but as the day progressed, the cramps worsened. She had already saturated two of the pads she brought with her. She stopped in the restroom to put on the last pad in her purse. When she stood up, she grew dizzy and lightheaded. She went to Martha's office to let her know she needed to go to the ER because she thought she might be having a miscarriage.

"I didn't know you were pregnant. I just thought you were putting on a few pounds."

"I was keeping it a secret, but now it's no longer a secret because I'm cramping and bleeding. Can you find someone to cover for me?"

"Not sure I can with this blizzard…Take some Motrin, that will help with the cramping."

"I'm afraid it will hurt the baby."

"If you are having a miscarriage, it is foolish to worry about hurting a fetus with Motrin."

Rachel teared up unexpectedly. Suddenly it was real that she might lose this pregnancy. "I really need to go. Please find someone."

Rachel walked back to the unit with tears in her eyes. She was in pain, the contractions in her abdomen were worsening. She started rounding on the second-shift patients. After one patient, Betty, one of the techs noticed some drops of blood on the floor seeping out between Rachel's pant legs, touched her on the shoulder, and told her.

Rachel whispered, "Can you see if anyone has an extra pad? I just used my last one." She gripped her abdomen, cried out, and fainted. Her head cracked on the floor as she fell.

Tamika called 911. As Rachel regained consciousness, Betty got a pillow for her head, started an IV, took her vital signs, and gave her oxygen. Rachel moaned in pain and held her lower abdomen.

Tamika put a cool washcloth on her head and said tenderly, "You're going to be okay. We called an ambulance. Is there anyone you would like me to call?"

Rachel heard Darnell yelling that he needed to get off the machine and shook her head. She knew that Darnell knew.

The ambulance arrived and as they lifted Rachel onto the stretcher with the IV and oxygen, Ms. Leggett appeared at her side. She placed a warm hand on Rachel's forehead. "I guess you weren't kidding when you told me you didn't feel well. Call me when you're ready to return to work."

Chapter 43

Darnell had awakened earlier that morning in Rachel's bed and smiled. He felt so full. He remembered the previous evening and the feeling of Rachel's skin next to his. He longed for her to be there beside him. He looked out the window, saw the blizzard, and wondered how the drive had been for Rachel earlier that morning. He wished dialysis units had snow days like schools, then he and Rachel could have cuddled in bed all morning. It was light outside when he drove to dialysis, but the snow swirled, and it was difficult to see the road. He inched along, arriving at the dialysis unit forty-five minutes late. He worried that his tardiness would throw off the dialysis schedule. But, when he arrived, he discovered several patients sitting in the waiting room. The blizzard had disrupted the entire dialysis schedule, and he'd still have to wait an hour for his chair.

The chatter in the waiting room concerned the blizzard. Blizzards have a way of bringing people to snuggle together, even dialysis patients in a waiting room. The patients shared stories around the circle as if they were telling stories over a campfire.

Darnell finally got on the machine and dialysis was going smoothly. Joe Fiorelli and J.R. babbled together. Their jokes and stories got on Darnell's nerves. Darnell thought, *I don't know which of the two of them is a bigger chatterbox. Whoever thought that putting those two talking heads together was a good idea?*

He saw Rachel walk into the unit from Ms. Leggett's office. She had tears in her eyes. Her face was pale, her eyebrows knitted together, and she had her hand over her lower abdomen. He watched intently as she tried to take care of a patient and gasped when he saw her collapse and heard her head crack on the floor. Betty and Tamika rushed to take care of her. He turned to J.R. and shouted, "Oh my God! I need to get off this machine and take care of her. J.R., what's the emergency take-off procedure? What do I do first?"

"Darnell, get a hold of yourself. You can't help her."

Darnell's stomach churned. This was the worst thing that he had ever seen. He hadn't known it was possible to feel so much anxiety and pain for another person.

"Are you hoping to give her some mouth-to-mouth resuscitation?" J.R. grinned, "Maybe we could take turns?"

"Stop it J.R.! That isn't funny!"

"Don't get your panties in a twist. We all love Rachel. She's going to be okay. If you got off the machine right now, you'd just add to the commotion."

Darnell looked directly at J.R., his face filled with worry. "What if she dies?"

"Darnell, get a grip. You lost more blood than that with your dialysis accident. I'm sure she'll be okay."

"She needs my help."

"Darnell, you'll be useless to help anyone if you don't get a good dialysis treatment today. Today's Friday. Did you know that most dialysis patients die on the weekend with an extra non-dialysis day thrown into the mix? You need to stay and finish your treatment."

"How'd you become a dialysis expert?"

"I've been on dialysis since you were in junior high. I know more than I pretend to know."

Darnell watched the ambulance carry Rachel away and sank into a black pit of anxiety. He suspected that Rachel was having a miscarriage but didn't know anything more about that or her risk of dying. He wondered if their lovemaking the night before caused it and was sick with worry and guilt.

He had never feared for another person so much in his entire life. The last two hours on the machine lasted for eternity. He fidgeted and watched the clock. He couldn't keep his legs still nor focus on any of the conversations in the unit. When he finally got off the machine, he was on a mission to get to the hospital. He gathered his blanket and possessions and quickly walked out of the unit into the cold white world. The wind blew the snow sideways, stinging his face. He noticed something peculiar on his beeline to his car. A body lying in the snow next to a car in the handicapped lane. He ran to the body and realized it was Mr. Freeman. "Oh fuck!" He saw Mr. Freeman's lower leg displaced at a right angle to the rest of his leg. The snow was already blanketing him.

Darnell bent over. "Mr. Freeman, are you okay? What happened?"

"I was standing next to my car door when my leg collapsed beneath me."

"Are you in pain?"

"Funny, I don't really feel anything but cold. I usually don't feel much in my legs because of the neuropathy."

Mr. Freeman was obese and walked slowly with a cane. He didn't have much strength. Darnell wanted to get him out of the cold but didn't think he could get him into a wheelchair. He pulled off his own coat to cover Mr. Freeman, rolled up his blanket and placed it under Mr. Freeman's head for a pillow.

"I'll get some help. I'll be right back." He ran into the unit and shouted to the secretary to call an ambulance for Mr. Freeman who broke his leg. He yelled so loudly that everyone in the unit heard. He ran to Ms. Leggett who had her reading glasses on, a syringe in her hand, and was slowly and painstakingly trying to figure out which patient got which medication.

"Can I use the fleece blankets in the gift bags for Mr. Freeman? The chill factor out there is sixteen below zero. I'm afraid to move him because his leg looks bad."

Ms. Leggett looked at Darnell and shook her head. "I'm only authorized to give those blankets to new patients."

Darnell grumbled. "I'm thinking United Dialysis Associates would be more concerned about letting a patient freeze to death in the parking lot."

"He's not going to freeze to death. The ambulance will be here in a few minutes."

The secretary ran in to inform them that the ambulance would be delayed because of the blizzard.

Ms. Leggett waved the syringe in her hand. "Go help yourself to the blankets. I'll send Tamika out to help once she finishes getting that patient off the machine."

When he returned to Mr. Freeman, he saw J.R. and Joe kneeling beside him, talking with him and telling him how awful his leg looked. Darnell took charge. "We need to get him to the waiting room where it's warm. The ambulance is delayed because of the blizzard. Maybe we can put some blankets underneath him and drag him over the snow into the unit. Luckily, the path to the waiting room is flat and there aren't any steps."

Darnell was afraid that one blanket wouldn't be able to hold Mr. Freeman's weight, so he put three blankets together. The wind bit Darnell's cheeks and his cold hands were getting stiff. "It's freezing out here. We need to hurry." *He's in so much danger. What if he gets frostbite or loses that leg? He's so big and heavy. What if we can't get him into the waiting room?* "Joe, can you hold his leg as J.R. and I roll him on to the blankets?" Joe created a sling to hold his leg up so it wouldn't get jostled as they turned and moved him. It was painstaking, slow work as they carefully rolled him onto the blankets. Mr. Freeman tried to help as much as he could while Joe protected his broken ankle. Slowly and deliberately, inch-by-inch, they pulled the blankets carrying Mr. Freeman across the snow-covered parking lot. They asked him frequently how he was doing and if they were hurting him. Luckily, the handicapped parking spaces were close to the front door. As more patients got off their machines, they gathered around to help, but most were too frail to be of any assistance. Some gave their coats and scarves to keep Mr. Freeman warm. Someone gave Darnell gloves when he saw his bare hands. Those who couldn't help, watched and cheered them on.

Tamika sprinted out of the unit pushing a wheelchair. They told her they wouldn't know how to lift Mr. Freeman onto the wheelchair and were afraid they might hurt him. Tamika agreed and encouraged them. "Only a few yards remaining." Tamika turned to go back to the unit. "Everyone is coming off the machines at once, and Betty and I need to tell Ms. Leggett which patients need which meds before they get off. I don't think she's passed meds on a dialysis patient since the turn of the century."

They slid Mr. Freeman through the automatic doors and into the waiting room. They used the blankets to pull him to a seated position against one of the chairs. The patients worked as a team. They removed all the snow-covered blankets and jackets that had been thrown on top of him. The UDA blankets were in shreds, so they just tossed them in the garbage. The secretary brought Mr. Freeman a cup of hot broth while Darnell went to pilfer a few more dry fleece blankets from the gift bags. He was so relieved that they had brought him to safety. None of the patients wanted to go home until the ambulance arrived. They sat around chatting with Mr. Freeman and each other. The secretary asked if he wanted her to call his wife.

"Yes, please. We were planning to leave tomorrow morning to go to Florida to visit our daughter. My wife is going to be so disappointed; she's been packing all afternoon. Tell her I'm in no pain and I'll call her from the hospital as soon as I know anything. Please tell her not to drive anywhere in this blizzard."

Anthony Fiorelli burst in. "I've never seen such a blizzard. Those roads are treacherous."

Joe stood. "Tony, you need to move your car, we're waiting for an ambulance to come for Mr. Freeman."

Anthony looked at Mr. Freeman's leg. "Ooh, that looks bad."

"I fell in the snow and your father helped rescue me."

"That's my dad." Anthony looked around. "Is Rachel working today? Perhaps I can give her a ride home? I hate to see anyone driving in this mess."

No one said a word.

After a long moment, Darnell said curtly. "She's not here." Darnell saw a flicker of disappointment cross Anthony's face.

Sirens blared and the ambulance arrived. The patients in the waiting room watched and clapped as the paramedics loaded Mr. Freeman onto the emergency stretcher and drove away.

- Chapter 44 -

Darnell's drive to the ER two miles away was painstakingly slow in the blizzard.

When he arrived, he asked the front desk receptionist for Rachel Rosen.

"Are you family?"

"Yes."

The receptionist did a double take. "What's your name?"

"Darnell Johnson."

The receptionist left and returned a few minutes later. "Come on back." She pressed a buzzer, opening the door to the entrance of the ER. "She's in Bay Five."

Darnell pushed aside the curtain to Bay Five and found Rachel lying on her side on the cot weeping. He started crying at the sight of her tears. He kissed her on the forehead, sat on the chair and held her hand. A unit of blood dripped through an IV in her arm. "Leif is gone, isn't he?"

Rachel rolled onto her back. "They took me to the OR and did an emergency D&E. Leif's head was stuck in my cervix, so they had to crush his head to get him out. They wrapped his tiny body in a blanket so I could hold him and say goodbye. He fit in the palm of my hand. He had perfect, tiny little fingers and toes. He was alive and kicking this morning and now he's gone."

Darnell wept. Through his tears he kept saying, "I'm sorry, so, so, sorry."

Darnell held her face in his hands. "When I saw you pass out in the dialysis unit, I was afraid I'd lose you forever."

Rachel shook her head. "I wasn't planning on dying. My

life has suddenly become exciting with you in it. When I heard you yell in the dialysis unit, I felt your love."

"You won't believe this though. Shortly after I arrived, police came to arrest me. Since the new anti-abortion law, every woman with vaginal bleeding is a suspect in an attempted abortion. My doctor yelled at the police, telling them that it was none of their business. I don't know what happened after that because they rushed me to the OR."

He asked tentatively, "Do you think having sex last night killed him? I never wanted to hurt Leif."

"If having sex could harm a fetus, I would have pushed you away no matter how much I wanted you."

Darnell hid his face in her abdomen. "I thought it was my fault."

She put her hands on his head and used his dreadlocks to gently pull his face to hers. "The miscarriage just happened. It's not your fault. It's part of life."

She started crying again. "I'll never be able to tell Leif about the first time I felt him move."

Darnell remembered hearing the sound her head made when it hit the floor and asked if they checked her head. She asked him through her tears, "Are you thinking that I've really lost it?"

"No. You cracked your head on the floor when you passed out. Does it hurt?"

"My head is killing me; I shouldn't be able to feel anything with all the drugs they gave me."

Darnell asked to speak to the ER doctor overseeing Rachel's care. He told her of the crack that reverberated through the dialysis unit when her head hit the floor. The doctor thanked him and had Rachel sit up so she could examine her head. She checked her pupils, her muscle strength, and her reflexes. The only abnormal finding was a large tender lump at the back of her head. The doctor told Rachel that on exam everything looked fine, but she still wanted to check a head CT to make sure there wasn't any bleeding inside her skull. "The CT may take a while because we're backed up in radiology. An awful leg fracture arrived a short time ago."

As they were waiting for the CT scan, Darnell told Rachel that he thought the leg fracture person could be Mr. Freeman. He told her about finding him on the ground next to his car and then using UDA fleece blankets to drag him to the waiting room.

"How in the world did those flimsy blankets pull him in?"

"We used three blankets. The parking lot was covered with snow, so that part was smooth going. J.R. and Joe Fiorelli helped me pull him in, but we nearly froze ourselves trying to save him."

"Joe Fiorelli was out in the snow helping?"

"He carried Mr. Freeman's leg in the sling. J.R. and Joe made quite the rescue team. Mr. Freeman said he didn't do anything or slip on anything. His leg just collapsed while he was standing next to the car."

Rachel's voice grew stern. "That's why we always nag everyone about controlling their phosphorus. After being on dialysis for a few years with a high phosphorus, people's bones become fragile, riddled with holes like Swiss cheese."

"I guess I better not pick up a pepperoni pizza on my way home tonight."

"You got that right. Can you check if it is really Mr. Freeman? Maybe we can visit him while we're waiting?"

"I'll go and investigate, but there is no way I'm pushing your cart to see Mr. Freeman. You need to rest. Your body has been through a lot today. Besides, I thought we were keeping our relationship secret."

He arrived at the nurse's station just in time to see them wheeling Mr. Freeman on a cart to surgery. Mr. Freeman noticed him and yelled. "There's Darnell. He is the one who saved me this afternoon."

Darnell waved to him and said, "I hope your surgery goes well tonight."

He returned to Bay Five as the radiology technician wheeled Rachel away for the head CT. He turned on the TV and saw that there had been twenty car accidents on the roads tonight, but the blizzard was moving to the east and the area was clearing.

When Rachel returned, he turned the TV off and told her the blizzard was clearing. Within minutes she dozed off. He sat on the metal chair next to the cart, lay his head on her chest and fell sound asleep.

Eventually, the nurse arrived to tell them that the CT was normal, the second unit of blood had finished, and Rachel could go home. She gave Rachel her home-going instructions and told her to avoid sex for six weeks until her uterus healed. Rachel and Darnell looked at each other and frowned.

"Can I drive you home?"

"I'm counting on it."

"I'm hoping you need me to stay with you tonight."

Rachel squeezed his hand. "I'm counting on that too."

Darnell pushed the wheelchair out of the ER into the frigid night. Rachel wore her sweater and coat but had to wear ER pajama pants home. The newly fallen snow sparkled like a million stars under the parking lot lights as the snow crunched under the wheelchair and Darnell's boots.

He was embarrassed when they arrived at his car. "I am sorry for this garbage can on wheels. I managed to clean my apartment a few months ago, but I only think of cleaning this car when I'm driving it, and then it's not the right time. Had I known I'd be driving you home today, I would have stayed up all night last night cleaning it out.

"Really, instead of our Hanukkah celebration?"

"No, I wouldn't trade last night for anything in the world."

When they arrived at Rachel's house, Darnell cooked them both scrambled eggs and toast before they fell asleep in each other's arms.

- Chapter 45 -

Darnell stayed with Rachel for a few days after her miscarriage, cooking her meals and playing gin rummy with her. She usually beat him in gin rummy, but he would remind her that he beat her in the game of Dreidel.

Rachel taunted him, "I know you won't admit it, but I won that game too. You're a loser across the board."

Darnell took her out for short walks in the white fairyland. Every day he'd start a fire in her fireplace, and they would discuss Leif and the miscarriage. Sometimes Rachel cried, other times they sat in companionable silence watching the flames. Rachel was surprised to be experiencing such grief. She hadn't even wanted the pregnancy. She kept repeating, "I should be relieved that I don't have to be a single mom."

"You wouldn't have been a single mom. I would have been with you every step of the way." On hearing that, Rachel snuggled closer to him.

Rachel returned to work the following week, filled with anxiety. She felt shame for hemorrhaging and passing out in the unit in front of everyone. She had failed to maintain her image as a competent professional. In full view of patients and staff, she had become the patient, helpless and dependent. She didn't know how people would react when they saw her again or if they would trust her with their care.

She needn't have been afraid though. Both patients and staff hugged her and welcomed her back to the unit. Some offered condolences about the miscarriage. She thanked them all for taking such good care of her and saving her life.

Work settled back into a routine, but life didn't feel normal. When she was home alone, she mourned and cried. It took weeks for her to absorb the reality that she had lost the pregnancy. Grief blindsided her, especially when she hadn't wanted to be pregnant to begin with. She was grateful she had only window-shopped baby furniture, toys, and clothes. It would have been worse if she had to look at all the baby items she had bought and be reminded that little Leif would never use them. Rachel returned the maternity and baby development books to the library and resumed reading nursing journals and novels. She remembered two friends who had suffered miscarriages previously and wrote them letters describing her own miscarriage and apologized for not seeing their pain.

On a gray December day when large snow flurries melted on the sidewalks, and Christmas decorations and lights festooned most homes and stores, Rachel bundled up in her coat, hat, and gloves to visit Miriam, Steve's mother, to let her know about the miscarriage. She parked her car in front of the familiar house and felt a twinge of sadness. She had spent her adolescence in this house. As she climbed the front steps, it occurred to her that this was the first time she had ever come through the front door. In the past, she'd barge in the back door to the kitchen, where she usually found Miriam cooking something delicious.

She rang the doorbell, expecting to see Miriam's face, but was met by a nurse's aide who explained to her that Miriam was now in hospice and Steve's dad was working. Even though Rachel had known the last-ditch chemotherapy wasn't working, her stomach dropped when she discovered Miriam in a hospital bed that monopolized the living room. *I should have been here for her.*

The room was stuffy and hot. Rachel quickly removed her outer garments. Odors of bleach and disinfectant assaulted her nose, but underneath those smells, Rachel detected hints of stool, urine, and a faint powdered cheese smell that reminded her of former dying patients. Rachel saw the outlines of

Miriam's shrunken and bony body under the sheets. Her cheeks were sunken, and her skull bones prominent. Miriam's cracked lips were moving, but she seemed to be sleeping. The aide went to the dining room to play with her cell phone as Rachel sat on the stuffed chair next to Miriam's bed and watched her labored breathing.

She remembered the living room's former elegance with a couch, loveseat, and chairs creating a cozy conversation area. Two stuffed chairs adjacent to the hospital bed and the painting of Jerusalem at sunrise on the wall across from the bay window were the only remnants of the former living room. Miriam's living room had become a dying room. A suction machine stood ready at a table next to her bed. The credenza was piled with medication bottles, boxes of rubber gloves, piles of disposable under pads, a bedpan, and boxes of too-thettes for moistening Miriam's dry mouth. The over-the-bed table held a phone, a box of Kleenex, a juice box with a straw, and an applesauce container with the foil peeled back.

The oxygen tubing that should have gone into Miriam's nose was askew at the side of her cheek. Rachel gently placed it back into her nose before taking Miriam's wrist in her hand.

Miriam's watery eyes opened. "Oh, it's you...I prayed to see you one last time."

"I wanted to see you too. How are you doing?"

Miriam replied in a weak and raspy voice that came in broken phrases, "Dying is boring...tedious...the thought of death once scared me...now my days are spent waiting for Hashem to call me home." She had to catch her breath between phrases. Rachel wondered at the wisdom of telling her about the miscarriage at this point, but she just blurted it out, "I had a miscarriage. I'm sorry. I had hoped to give you a chance to hold a grandchild before you passed on."

Miriam touched Rachel's arm. "It's okay." She stopped

talking to catch her breath. "I'm sorry you had the miscarriage…not for myself but for you…I had two miscarriages between Stevie and Maxine…so much sorrow." She closed her eyes and was quiet for a long time.

Rachel couldn't tell if Miriam was dozing or remembering. She continued holding her hand, her chest tight with grief to be losing this kind woman who had been her surrogate mother. She had helped her with her first period, taught her how to cook, and encouraged her when she struggled in nursing school.

After a while, Miriam looked at Rachel. "I'm sorry you and Stevie broke up…The first I knew the two of you were having problems was Rosh Hashanah." She shook her head. "Stevie has lost his soul."

Miriam dozed off again. Rachel grabbed a Kleenex to tenderly wipe the dribble at the corner of her mouth. Rachel sat for a while; her heart lulled into silence by the rhythmic low rumble of the oxygen concentrator. She petted Miriam's hand, shaken by her impending loss. She gazed around the room and at the stairs leading to the second floor and remembered running up and down them with Steve and Maxine hundreds of times. *A different life. Who was that young woman?* Everything had changed. Her body, her relationships, her job, her faith, and the things that brought her joy. For many years she believed that she would be part of this family forever.

As she sat, she prayed for a peaceful death for Miriam, and prayed for Steve to find his soul again, realizing that this was the first time since she left him that it occurred to her to pray for him. Eventually, Rachel stood to say goodbye, knowing that this would be the last time she would ever see Miriam. With tears in her eyes, she kissed her on the forehead and told her she loved her. Miriam took a halting breath. "I love you too, Rachel."

Rachel bundled up to go into the cold and as she walked

down the front steps weeping, Maxine drove up the driveway. The two of them hugged for a long time and sobbed, wiping tears from each other's eyes. "How are you holding up?"

Maxine continued crying. "I can't eat. I can't do my work. I can't study. I hate watching her die. I'm losing her inch by inch. All she does is sleep and I can't get her to eat anything. She had so many friends. Now she refuses to see any of them. The only people she talks to now are people who aren't there."

Rachel put her hands on Maxine's shoulders and looked into her eyes. "Usually when a dying person starts talking to people not there, it means their time to die is close. I don't think it will be long now."

Rachel started crying again. "Your mom was always so kind to me. Her memory will always be a blessing."

Maxine looked away. "I wish I could help her."

Rachel sighed. "Me too. I think the only thing you can do is to tell her every day that you love her."

"I've missed you. I've felt so guilty about you and Steve splitting. I'm sorry I brought the ultrasound out on Rosh Hashanah."

"It's not your fault. Things hadn't been going well between us for months."

"How's your pregnancy progressing? Boy or girl?"

Rachel took a deep breath. "I miscarried a few weeks ago. It was a boy."

Maxine teared up. "I would have loved to have been an aunt to your baby."

"You'd have been the best."

Maxine told Rachel that she was almost finished with her degree in social work and still working as a waitress at Howard's Deli to support herself. They agreed to keep in touch and meet for lunch soon. Maxine promised to let her know when her mom passed.

Rachel often visited Elizabeth and Buckeye. Initially, she was surprised to discover Dr. Max Burnouf accompanying

Elizabeth on her daily walks. Eli didn't need her company anymore, but Rachel enjoyed their company. The friendship between Elizabeth and Max was welcoming and full of hospitality.

Occasionally, Elizabeth would invite Rachel over for Sunday dinners as Darnell continued to spend his Sunday afternoons at Mama's. (Neither Rachel nor Darnell wanted J.R. to know about their relationship.) Elizabeth's daughters and their boyfriends sometimes came to the Sunday dinners. Sunday afternoons at Elizabeth's house were characterized by bantering and laughing. Some afternoons were spent arguing over Becky and Joe's wedding preparations, other Sunday afternoons they hiked in the parks. During inclement weather they played board games.

- Chapter 46 -

It was New Year's Day, a non-dialysis day. A few staff were on call for emergencies which usually fell into one of two categories. The most common was fluid overload from dietary indiscretions. The other reason for emergency dialysis on holidays was for kidney transplants. Holidays are peak drunk driving days. Car accidents from drunk drivers kill otherwise healthy individuals, creating the perfect organ donor. It's rather macabre, but dialysis patients get their hopes up for a possible kidney transplant whenever holidays roll around.

Rachel spent New Year's Eve at Darnell's apartment. Neither were superstitious, but they wholeheartedly adhered to the New Year's Eve superstition that says, 'Who you kiss at midnight is the person you will be kissing for the rest of the year.' They still had three weeks to go before they could have sex again, but they were creative in finding alternate ways of loving each other and giving each other pleasure. They relished each other's company and couldn't keep their hands off each other.

Rachel and Darnell planned to have Shanita and her sons over for dinner. Beef brisket was roasting in the oven. Shanita and her sons weren't due to arrive for two hours, so Rachel and Darnell hung out. Music played on the stereo as Rachel sat on Darnell's lap, facing him and playing with his dreadlocks, braiding and unbraiding them as they bantered about everything on their hearts.

Darnell asked Rachel if she was in the habit of making New Year's Resolutions.

"Since I'm Jewish, I celebrate New Year's twice a year.

You'd think making resolutions twice a year would make me twice as good. The problem is, I usually forget my resolutions after a week or so, and then I'm stuck with the same old fallible, flawed me."

Darnell nodded, "I've read that most resolutions fail in a matter of weeks.

"But people grow and change all the time. If it's not resolutions, what do you think causes people to change?"

"I think it's disappointments, suffering, and trials…those times when life isn't what you wanted or hoped it would be. In nature, seeds are broken in the dirt before they sprout into something new and alive."

"Now, that's poetic. However, people don't automatically become better with suffering. Sometimes they become bitter."

Darnell tilted his head. "I guess the secret lies in accepting the suffering as you walk through it. I was bitter for a long time. It's not easy. Almost dying changed me too. Things don't bother me like they used to."

Rachel touched his cheek. "Leif changed me. Because of him, I chose a different path. Grief over his loss is also changing me. I'm more aware of other people's pain."

Darnell kissed her. "Perhaps love is really the linchpin that changes people."

Rachel waxed philosophical as she continued to braid Darnell's dreadlocks. "The real question is, is it really a new year or just the day after yesterday?"

Darnell smiled. "Well, the earth, in its journey around the sun, was in the same place as it is right now a year ago." He stopped for a minute. "Hmmm. The earth may be taking the same old trip around the sun, but I'm not. Since last New Year's, I've returned to college, gotten beat up by cops, spent time in ICU where I almost died, and now you're here sitting on my lap."

Rachel nodded. "Yeah, my life has seen a lot of changes

since my last trip around the sun too. Let's take a walk along the lake to celebrate this new year together."

Darnell pretended to shiver. "Rachel, it's freezing out there. There's nothing to block the wind and the lake has already started to ice over. Stay here on my lap where we won't get frostbite."

Suddenly, the door to Darnell's apartment flew open, and Shanita walked in weeping uncontrollably. Clarence and Lester followed, holding hands, bewildered by their mother's tears. Darnell rushed to her and put his arms around her. She couldn't stop crying to tell Darnell what had happened.

He held her for a while. "What happened? Is Mama okay? What happened? What happened?"

"Mama wants you to come to the hospital right now."

"What happened to Mama?"

"Someone shot Will." Shanita wailed. "He's dead. They're keeping him on life support. Mama told the doctors that she wants you to receive Will's kidney."

Darnell collapsed to the floor weeping uncontrollably. "I don't want his kidney. I want Will alive. I don't want his kidney. I want my brother. I want my brother."

They held on to each other on the floor and wept. The twins and Rachel watched the scene as outsiders. They cried because those they loved were weeping. Rachel pulled the twins to her lap, hugging them. After an interminable amount of time, Rachel realized she needed to take charge.

She put the twins down and turned off the oven. "Time to head to the hospital. The sooner Darnell receives his brother's kidney, the better the chance of a good outcome."

Darnell was still crying, resistant. "I just want my brother alive."

Rachel knelt close to Darnell and touched the tattoo on his arm, the Japanese characters declaring, 'This moment only once.' "This is not the moment you would choose as the opportunity to get off dialysis, not the moment anyone would choose, but it's the moment given to you today, right now. You need to take it. You will never find such a perfect kidney match in your life. It will take a long time to grieve the loss of Will, but at least you will have a part of him inside you. Come on. Let's go."

They took two cars. Rachel drove Darnell, and Shanita followed in her car with the twins. Darnell rocked back and forth in his seat, hitting his forehead with his fist. "Why did I bail him out? I'm so stupid. It's my fault. All my fault. If he were still in jail, he'd be alive."

Rachel shook her head. "It isn't your fault. You bailed him out because you loved him and because you love Mama. It's not your fault."

Darnell put his head in his hands. "I hated Will's addiction. Sometimes I couldn't even look at him because I hated his addiction so much. It was a monster that swallowed him up. I could always fight him but lost every battle against his addiction. We were so close when we were younger. As we grew older, we fought a lot. Sometimes I'd be so angry that I would've killed him with my bare hands if I had the strength. Will started getting into drugs when he was fourteen. I don't know why I didn't. He was much more social than I was and had a lot of friends and things to do. My drug of choice was a good book. A perfect day for me was taking the RTA to the Cleveland Public Library. I got lost in the book stacks as my brother got lost smoking crack."

They pulled into the ER parking lot, and before they got out of the car, Rachel took his head in her hands and kissed him with her whole heart. "The next few months are going to be difficult, but like you were telling me right before Shanita arrived, lean into the pain and the sorrow even as you accept your brother's kidney. I know you'd rather have him alive than have his kidney, but this is what you have right now. Love will get us through."

The ER staff were awaiting them when they walked in. They ushered Darnell back for labs and testing, and directed Rachel, Shanita, and her twins to the waiting room. They were greeted by Mama and J.R., who had been sitting there for hours. They wept together as they waited. Mama told Shanita and Rachel through her tears that Will had gone a few weeks prior to have his kidneys tested. He wanted it to be a surprise for Darnell. They all started crying again. Mama asked Shanita if she wanted to pay her last respects to Will in the ICU. Shanita and Mama left to go to the ICU, leaving Rachel and J.R. to watch the twins.

Clarence and Lester were agitated, needing to be held. Rachel pulled Lester to her lap, and J.R. picked up Clarence. They sat next to each other on the stiff plastic chairs in the waiting room.

J.R. turned to Rachel, shaking his head. "I knew you drove Darnell home from dialysis that time, but how did you end up driving him here today?"

"I was sitting on Darnell's lap when Shanita arrived with the news."

J.R. did a double take. "What? You two together? Now I understand why Darnell got so upset when you passed out in dialysis." J.R. shook his head. "He was insane. He wanted to do the emergency take-off procedure and rush to save you."

Rachel smiled. "I know. I heard him yelling. We kept our relationship secret because I'd probably lose my job if I were caught dating one of my patients. Once Darnell gets this kidney though, he'll no longer be my patient, and we'll no longer have to hide our relationship."

J.R. patted his chest. "I don't think this old heart can take any more shocks today. Was the miscarriage Darnell's baby?"

"No, it was Steve Silverman's baby, my former fiancé. We broke up when he wanted me to get an abortion."

Rachel had started playing with Lester's dreadlocks absently as she spoke. Clarence reached over to Rachel and said, "Me too."

Rachel looked at J.R. "I think I've started something; you have to give Clarence a head massage."

J.R. laughed and started massaging Clarence's head. "So now that you're dating Darnell and I'm married to Ruby, you will be my daughter-in-law if the two of you get married. We'd be family. Connected in crazy ways. Outrageous."

"We were already connected in so many ways. However, don't expect any special treatment from me in the dialysis unit."

"You did a nice job of treating Darnell as just another patient…I'd never have guessed."

"Did you know Will? What happened?"

"I met Will for the first time when he moved in with Ruby and me. I didn't get much of a chance to know him. The moment he arrived; he was antsy to be with his old friends. Some nights he didn't come home, other nights he came home high. He stole Ruby's laptop. I know his family is grieving over him, remembering who he was. I'm sure at one time he was lovable, but I didn't like him. I wanted to beat him daily for all the aggravation he caused Ruby."

"Do you know what happened? Who shot him?"

"Someone called an ambulance from a drug house. When the ambulance arrived, they found his body on the floor, bleeding. No one else was around. He was still breathing, and his heart was beating when they brought him to the ER. They worked on him but couldn't save him. I suspect someone may have been afraid he would talk as part of a plea bargain. I know he was considering it. The police are investigating, but we may never know what really happened."

Darnell walked into the waiting room. "They drew my blood. They plan to do a special test in the OR to make sure my heart valves weren't damaged by the infection. They're doing extra studies on Will's blood to be sure he doesn't have any viruses to pass on to me or any other organ recipients. I had to sign a form that I was accepting an organ from a high-risk donor."

Rachel said, "Shanita and Mama are upstairs in the ICU, paying their final respects. I bet there's time left for you to go now if you wish."

"First, let me try to explain everything to Clarence and Lester." He sat on another chair and his nephews climbed on his lap. "Do you remember Uncle Will?"

They looked up at him with total trust and shook their heads.

"Will was my brother like you two are brothers. When we were little, we played together every day. We slept in the same bed. We were always a part of each other, but today he died. That's why I'm crying. But he left me his kidney, so I won't have to go to dialysis anymore. In fifteen minutes, I'll go to my last dialysis session, and then I'll go to surgery to have an operation to get Will's kidney. Afterwards I'll be in the hospital a few days, but after that, I'll come home and tell you all about it." He kissed and hugged them both, and they snuggled against him, not wanting him to go.

Rachel watched Darnell's gentleness and tenderness as he tried to explain the situation to his nephews and fell in love with him all over again. She knew they didn't understand a word of what he told them but suspected they would always remember his love for them.

When Darnell was ready to pay his last respects to his brother, he reluctantly put his nephews back into J.R. and Rachel's laps. "Now I have to go and thank Will for giving me his kidney and say goodbye." He had tears in his eyes.

Thirty minutes later, Mama, Shanita, and Darnell returned to the waiting room with tears in their eyes, and Darnell went for dialysis. Ruby announced that she had given permission to donate any other of Will's organs that were viable. Will had been shot in the head but was still breathing when he arrived at the hospital. They were hoping to transplant his heart, lungs, the other kidney, liver, and cornea. Ruby wept. "At least his death will bring life to other people who are suffering."

Rachel and the rest of his family went to the dialysis unit waiting room to sit with Darnell during his treatment. Only one person was allowed in at a time. After a few hours, a surgical nurse came to the dialysis unit to tell Darnell they were ready for him and directed the family members to the surgical waiting room on the third floor. The nurse told them that the surgery would last three to four hours. Before Darnell left, he gave everyone a hug: his mama, Shanita, J.R., his nephews again, and then Rachel. That last hug lasted the longest. He didn't want to let go of her, nor she him. Rachel, nervous, wished the surgery were over already.

Shanita announced she was going home to put her sons down for a nap. Rachel decided to go to Darnell's apartment to slice the beef brisket and bring it back with some rolls to make sandwiches. Her stomach was rumbling, and she thought Mama and J.R. would be hungry after the long day so far.

Rachel arrived at Darnell's apartment and discovered that even though she had turned the oven off, the meat had continued cooking in the warm oven and was now tender and falling apart. She tried to slice it, but Darnell's kitchen knives were duller than butter knives. She ended up tearing the beef apart with forks and adding the gravy. It would still make delicious sliders. As she walked out the door, she remembered that Darnell didn't bring clothes to wear in the hospital. She gathered his toothbrush and razor from the bathroom and went to his bedroom to gather some clothes. She tried to open the top drawer of his dresser, which still stuck. She pulled it hard, and once again the contents dumped on the floor. She whacked her forehead and exclaimed, "Not again!" As she gathered his clothes, she reminded herself to ask Darnell what the trick was to opening that drawer in the future. Darnell didn't own an overnight bag, so she used a grocery bag as a suitcase.

Rachel returned to the surgical waiting room to find J.R holding Mama as she wept. She kept saying over and over between her sobs, "I loved him so much. So many many hopes and dreams for his life." She looked into J.R.'s eyes. "Why didn't Jesus heal him? I prayed for him even when I wasn't praying. I tried so hard. I did everything I could."

J.R. kissed her on her head as he held her. "I don't know why he wasn't healed. Remember the psalm we read in church last week. I think the words were, 'The Lord is close to the broken hearted.' God weeps with you. I think He wanted Will to be healed more than you did"

J.R sighed. "Perhaps God shouldn't have given us so much free will."

Rachel's heart was filled with compassion for Ruby, for the tears in things, for the idea that God cried with us. After Ruby's tears quieted, she asked her this. "Did Darnell ever tell you what happened to him the night he almost died in the ICU while you prayed in the waiting room?

Ruby looked at up. "I know God granted him life."

"That schmuck. He promised to tell you. He spent that night while they were trying to save his life, and you were praying, on a park bench with Jesus. He felt no pain or anxiety, just peace. It changed him."

Ruby's weeping resumed. "Sometimes, like today with Will dying, I feel my prayers float in outer space unanswered, but here you tell me that Jesus was near to Darnell when he was dying and granted him life. I just hope Will knows God's peace now, which he couldn't find on earth."

Will's kidney started making urine during surgery the moment it was attached. The transplant team discharged

Darnell home from the hospital two days later. Darnell stayed with Rachel, his private duty nurse, for the first few weeks. She drove him to the hospital for follow-up testing until he could drive himself.

This time around Rachel enjoyed seeing Darnell's empty chair in the dialysis unit. It was soon filled by a young woman whose kidneys failed because of lupus. In characteristic fashion, J.R. took her under his wings, teaching her everything he knew or thought he knew. Rachel countered his sometimes misinformation with more accurate pamphlets and handouts. The one thing they both agreed wholeheartedly on was that she needed to get on the transplant list as soon as possible.

After a few weeks, Darnell came to visit his old friends in the dialysis unit. Everyone clapped when he walked in with a huge grin on his face. Patients and staff swarmed him, hugged him, and asked a million questions.

- Chapter 47 -

One January morning, as Rachel was drinking coffee and reading email, the doorbell rang. She opened the door to discover Steve standing there. He asked if he could have a word with her. The only time she had seen him since the day she moved out was across the synagogue at his mother's funeral.

She still had hot coffee in her pot and offered him a cup, preparing it as she knew he liked it with cream, a spoonful of sugar, and a dusting of cinnamon. She handed him the steaming mug and sat across from him at the kitchen table. "What's up?"

"Your patient, Daniel, will be receiving money from the city of Cleveland. They settled out of court because they didn't want the publicity."

Rachel groaned. "His name is Darnell."

"Whatever. Anyway, we settled for two hundred fifty thousand dollars."

Rachel smiled. "Wow. That's a lot of money. So that means you'll be receiving close to eighty thousand?"

He grinned. "All in a day's work. The money doesn't come to me though; it goes to my firm, but it's good for my career."

Rachel smiled. "Have you told him?"

"I called him today."

"I've been meaning to call you; I miscarried the day of the blizzard. It was a boy. That lets you off the hook for child support. They sent his tissues to the lab to be sure there weren't any genetic abnormalities that you'd need to be aware of, but everything came back normal."

"I know. Maxine told me. It would have been easier for you

if you had just had that abortion."

Rachel sighed. "I suppose an abortion would have been easier…but keeping the pregnancy changed my life. I would have learned to be a good mother."

Steve offered quietly, "I would have learned to be a good father too."

That comment stunned Rachel, and she wondered about his change of heart. She offered condolences on his mother's death. "I feel like I've lost my mother too. She was more mother to me than my own mother."

"That's not saying much. Your mom's mean."

"Yeah, I know." She took in a deep breath. "How are you doing with your mother's passing?"

Steve stared vacantly at the floor for a few long minutes as Rachel waited in the silence. "Maxine told me you visited my mom two days before she died. Thank you."

"I didn't do it for you. I did it for her. I did it for me. I wanted to tell her about the miscarriage. I would have visited her earlier and more often had I known she was so near to death."

"I know you loved her. I've been thinking a lot about everything. The real reason I came today is to ask you to come back home. I miss you. I'm sorry I took you for granted."

Rachel tilted her head and spoke sharply, "What happened to Kathy, your little Shikse? Are you planning to continue doing us both?"

"How'd you find out about her?"

"Remember…I saw you put your hand on her butt at that cocktail party a lifetime ago."

"We've broken up. She has a nice body, but she's hollow inside."

"A match made in Heaven."

Steve grimaced. "I've never known you to be so snarky before."

"I don't think you knew me at all."

Steve frowned and shook his head. "That's not true. I know you better than I know anyone else. I miss you…The house is empty without you."

"There's another man in my life."

Steve did a double-take. "Is it Anthony? He's always talking about how kind you are and how you helped his father. He seems smitten with you."

"No."

"You found someone so quickly? Rebound romances don't last. Don't throw away all the years we shared together."

"You're the one who threw those years away."

He mumbled, cracking his knuckles. "I was stupid. I promise to be faithful from here on out."

"It's too late for promises." Rachel rose to usher him to the door, but Steve didn't take the hint and sat at her kitchen table looking dejected. Rachel resisted the urge to comfort him and carried his coat to the door, signaling that she had already closed the door to their relationship. "The past is gone."

He rose slowly and reluctantly put on his coat.

After she closed the door behind him, she leaned against it for a few minutes, processing his visit. She poured herself the remaining coffee and sat at the kitchen table for a long time. She congratulated herself on her decisiveness with Steve, but when she remembered their years together, she questioned her resolve. Everything about him was so familiar. His mannerisms, his smell. *Is the past really gone? The years spent with him are still a part of me, part of who I am.* His words and familiar presence had awakened something she thought had died. She wondered about the connection she still felt to him and wondered if he had really changed. She realized that if there was anything she knew about life so far, it is that change is the only constant.

There was a time in her life when she felt it crucial to marry a Jewish man, someone who shared her traditions like

Steve did. They were in the same Bar Mitzvah class together, for God's sake. She wondered if, in choosing Darnell, she'd be walking away from a part of herself. Would Darnell encourage their children to become Bar or Bat Mitzvahs? Would he attend synagogue with her? So many questions and gray areas. She didn't like the gray areas. She realized that she and Darnell had many things to hammer out. As she pondered further, she remembered Steve's abuse and control. She remembered the times he caused her to doubt herself and how lonely she felt with him at times. Then she considered Darnell. *I love him. He's the kindest person I ever knew. I trust him. Even though he isn't Jewish, he's a mensch. We'll figure out the faith piece together. God is bigger than any single religion.*

- Chapter 48 -

Elizabeth retired from her work as a NP in the dialysis unit. She was losing her mojo, finding it difficult to concentrate. She worried that she would miss something critical and harm a patient. The fatigue was overwhelming and there were days she fell asleep in her office at work. Her appetite wasn't what it used to be, and she was losing weight for the first time in her life.

In the nephrology field there aren't set criteria as to the best time to start dialysis. Each person is unique. Many nephrologists wait for the patient to say, "I'm ready." But that's a fuzzy line to draw. Some people are never ready. Failing kidneys provide an uneven journey with good and bad days. The good days convince a person that they still have time before dialysis. Some research suggests that patients who start dialysis earlier live longer, but the converse argument to that is that they just spend more time on dialysis than patients who start dialysis later. Max (and her new nephrologist) encouraged Elizabeth to start dialysis, encouraging her that she'd be able to return to work once she felt better. She resisted. She didn't want to return to work. She wanted to avoid starting dialysis. Max understood her reluctance to return to work. He was planning his own retirement. Nephrology is a difficult specialty; interesting and challenging but under-appreciated by patients. Patients don't bring gifts to their nephrologist when they start dialysis like they do for cardiac surgeons after heart surgery and oncologists after chemotherapy as gratitude for saving their lives. Perhaps it's because kidney disease is silent, insidious, the cures limited, and a life on dialysis arduous.

Max told Elizabeth, "I understand returning to work isn't going to motivate you to start dialysis. Here's another angle: I know you like the thought of losing weight, but we both know that you are becoming malnourished. That's probably the most important reason for you to start dialysis. Now that we're together, I want to have you around for a few years."

"Max, I can't explain it. I wish I had followed my diet better and exercised more regularly…you know…all the things we always told our patients to do; then I wouldn't be facing the prospect of dialysis.

"Perhaps a better diet would have helped for a while, maybe not. It's not good medicine to blame a person for getting sick; worse medicine for a person to blame themselves for getting sick. We don't have control over the things that really make a difference, like the genes a person is born with or aging."

"Yeah, the control we think we have is an illusion."

"But you do have control over when to start dialysis."

"I know, and I'm not ready."

These theoretical conversations about the timing of the start of dialysis went on for weeks until Max enlisted Elizabeth's daughters again. They arrived together one Sunday afternoon and were aghast to discover Elizabeth choosing a playlist for her funeral. She told them that she didn't want a funeral per se, but a party for everyone after a short service. She was thinking along the lines of a traditional Irish wake.

The conflagration that ensued made her daughters' earlier confrontation feel like nursery school story time.

"Mom, you promised us," Becky bemoaned. "You promised to be around for our wedding. How can you be so stubborn?"

Lauren told her, "You aren't yourself; your personality has changed. You never want to do anything anymore. Your skin is gray and your breath smells."

Once again, her daughters prevailed, and Elizabeth made the appointment to get a graft put in her arm to start dialysis. Elizabeth started dialysis in the same dialysis unit where Rachel worked. This arrangement was just temporary because Max and Eli were on the waiting list for home dialysis training. Even though Max was a doctor, the home care nurses required him to go through home dialysis training like everyone else. Though he had written thousands of dialysis prescriptions in his career, he had never set up a dialysis machine nor trouble-shooted alarms or problems. Elizabeth and Max had decided together upon short dialysis sessions of two hours daily for six days a week, which was doable. During dialysis sessions, they planned to catch up on their reading, play games, or watch movies together.

Elizabeth requested that Rachel do the honors of inserting her dialysis needles for the first time. Buckeye sat in quiet attention next to Elizabeth's chair as Rachel tenderly took Elizabeth's arm and whispered to her that she loved her before inserting the needles. Ms. Leggett came out of her office to give Elizabeth a 'welcome to dialysis bag' complete with a flimsy fleece blanket. She spent more time by her chair than she had spent with any other new patient. In fact, everyone in the unit spent time at her chair. She was queen of the dialysis unit during the weeks she waited for home dialysis training. So much for boundaries and not showing favoritism to patients.

- Chapter 49 —

The first few months after his transplant, Darnell found himself in a liminal space. He relished the pleasure of urinating again and eating his favorite foods. Feeling normal felt extraordinary. He loved the luxury of more time; three extra days to fill as he chose each week. He increased his hours at the Cash Flash Pawn shop and took on more coursework. He'd be ready to start student teaching the following spring. The settlement money also added to his sense of well-being. Money for a future. The court refunded the bail money, and he repaid Howard the pawn money in exchange for the keys and registration for Rusty.

But with his good fortune came the catastrophe of losing his brother. He had a difficult time reconciling the two realities. It wasn't just grief; it was grief smothered in guilt. He kept thinking of things he could have done or said that would have kept Will clean and kept him alive. He thought of angles he could have tried and missed opportunities. He'd lacked the skills and knowledge to help him. He lamented bailing him out of jail relentlessly as waves of guilt roiled his heart. He dreamt about his brother often, and when he awakened to remember he was gone, his eyes filled with tears. He wondered if Will was still Will somewhere. His mother had raised him on resurrection stories, but his faith dissolved in his grief.

His eyes filled with tears at random unexpected times, like when he passed an outdoor basketball court or drove past the bar where they stayed after 'last call,' the day he bailed Will out of jail. His nephews reminded him constantly of the kinship he and Will had shared when they were little. He remembered the good times, the times before his brother's drug addictions.

His main solace was seeing Rachel when she got off work. Rachel listened and comforted him as he processed his grief and guilt. He parked the settlement money in a savings account as he considered the opportunities it provided. He wanted to use part of the settlement for a down payment on a house in Cleveland Heights for Shanita and the boys. The mortgage payments would be similar to her current rent pay- ments. Though he hadn't abandoned his dream of teaching in the inner city, he knew intimately the Cleveland school sys- tem's shortcomings and wanted his nephews to have every educational opportunity for success. Rachel, Darnell, and Shanita spent Sunday afternoons exploring open houses. They were especially intrigued by some older duplexes and imagined a future for their families living side by side.

In the stratosphere of those days, they heard talk of a novel coronavirus causing a possible pandemic on the other side of the world. Rachel read everything she could about it, wondering if it would spread to America. Darnell meanwhile readied Rusty for the first balmy spring day, regaling Rachel with the joys of spring motorcycle riding.

- Chapter 50 -

On March 16, the Governor of Ohio declared a Covid lockdown. Covid 19, which had started with fifteen cases in the US the previous month, now had over 82,000 cases and over 16,000 deaths.

Rachel called Darnell that afternoon. "Darnell, we can't see each other until Covid is gone."

"What??? I thought we were partners."

"Haven't you heard about the Governor declaring a lockdown?"

"Of course. But he didn't mean us, just the general public. I'm happy to avoid strangers."

"Darnell, the virus isn't that smart. It can't tell lover from stranger. It just spreads from one human to another. I'm terrified of giving you Covid. I'm afraid it might kill you."

Darnell wasn't happy with this new turn of events and took it personally, feeling like Rachel was pushing him away. "The virus won't kill me. Not seeing you will kill me." He hung up on her.

Rachel called him right back to reassure him that the lockdown would just last a few weeks. She told him of the first SARS pandemic. It was eliminated with simple public health measures of quarantine, isolation, and testing.

Darnell wasn't that easily mollified. He thought she picked a terrible time to separate from him, on the cusp of spring, especially with the novelty of a pandemic. What an adventure to experience together. As he stewed in his apartment, a nurse from the transplant office called and instructed him to quarantine more than the average joe because the anti-rejection medications for his kidney transplant suppressed his immune system. He took a deep breath. *Okay. I hope it only lasts two weeks.*

Things changed quickly in Ohio.

Cleveland State shut down for a few weeks before switching to online classes.

The Cash Flash Pawn shop closed.

The twins' daycare center closed.

Darnell became nanny to his nephews, so Shanita could continue working. He struggled to complete his coursework with toddlers clamoring for his attention and with an unreliable internet to boot. His nephews wore him out, and he ran out of ideas for their entertainment in his tiny apartment. The Children's Museum, the Cleveland Zoo, public libraries, and playgrounds all shut down. In desperation, Darnell allowed the twins to run back and forth in the hallways of the apartment building and play hide and seek using the elevator until his neighbors complained about the racket. He capitulated and let his nephews watch too much TV.

- Chapter 51 -

Rachel found her life upended also. Covid was new; no one knew how it spread or how it wreaked such havoc in the human body. Testing was limited and it took weeks to get results. Rachel struggled with anxiety. Several dialysis technicians and nurses resigned because they feared bringing Covid home to their families. She was glad she wasn't pregnant anymore and wondered if she would have continued working if she were still pregnant. Leif would have been near-term.

Patients were separated six feet apart from one another in the waiting room, and their dialysis chairs were positioned beyond conversation distance. Masks and social distancing put an end to friendly dialysis conversations. Fear reigned. Everyone became a possible agent of infection, so patients kept their distance and waved. J. R. became serious and morose. The nor- mal background chatter of the dialysis unit disappeared. The beeping of the dialysis machine alarms punctuated the som- ber silence. Rachel and the other staff dressed in full gowns, masks, and face shields. Rachel sweated in the gowns and squinted through the steamed face shield to draw up meds and read the dials on the dialysis machines.

Patients became abusive, blaming the dialysis staff for the restrictions…as if they made up the virus just to tor- ture patients. It was difficult for many to believe an invisible virus was real. She knew they felt scared, isolated, and alone because she felt scared, isolated, and alone, walking a tight- rope between wanting to comfort her patients and protecting herself from the virus. She had read reports of nurses con- tracting Covid and dying. Once again Rachel asked herself the perennial question, "Am I cut out to be a nurse?" This question was a little more nuanced this time around though. She wondered if nursing was worth dying for.

Some patients stopped showing for treatment when they heard authorities telling people to stay home. Rachel called the missing patients to tell them that the chance of 'no dialysis' killing them was certain, but Covid was full of unknowns. It was during these phone calls that Rachel first heard conspiracy theories about Covid. Some patients believed the government made the virus up to control the populace or withheld the cures to kill people. She tried to counter their misinformation with what she knew, always reminding patients that everyone was flying blind. There were so many unknowns....

Her usual eight-hour workday stretched into a twelve-hour workday because of the staggered shifts designed to keep the patients socially distanced and the exodus of the staff. Remaining staff were often required to quarantine for exposures leaving an even smaller skeleton crew staffing the dialysis unit. Some weeks Rachel clocked in over eighty hours to cover for staffing shortages.

Even with the extreme precautions, some patients still contracted Covid. Many were hospitalized, never to return. The patients who managed to survive often suffered a new layer of infirmity. On top of that, a batch of new dialysis patients arrived. These were people who survived Covid, but not before Covid killed their kidneys. They had no preparation for dialysis and arrived with permcaths and in shock at how their lives had been upended by a virus.

Joe Fiorelli was the first patient to die, and Rachel felt his death keenly. She had taken so much pleasure in his progress and adaptation to dialysis. She loved his 'can do' attitude and desire to be useful. His death felt like a failure. She sent sympathy cards to Joe's wife and Anthony. Rachel and J.R. cried together six feet apart, afraid to touch and hug. J.R. and Joe had become fast friends. Joe had started looking forward to his dialysis treatments so he could hang out with J.R. Before Covid they spent their dialysis treatments bantering back and forth and solving the world's problems.

After grueling days, Rachel stumbled home to an empty house, too tired to read or eat. Some days she just collapsed onto her bed. She missed Darnell. The cold, empty fireplace mirrored the loneliness in her heart. Instead of cuddling and telling each other stories in the evenings, Rachel and Darnell moaned and complained about their days over FaceTime.

During their evening phone calls, when she complained, Darnell encouraged her to quit her job. "I can support you with the settlement money. You're risking your health for patients who don't love you like I do, who don't appreciate everything you do for them."

"Who's going to take care of them? I can't leave now. Everyone's abandoning them."

When Darnell complained about caring for his nephews, Rachel would say, "You're risking your life taking care of your nephews. Shanita is exposed to Covid in the nursing home."

"Who's going to take care of them? My sister needs to work. I can't abandon them. They're my nephews."

"I guess we're both stuck."

Darnell countered with, "Since we're both stuck, I think you can stop worrying about giving me Covid and come over and see me. I want to run my hands through your hair."

"No, seeing me doubles your risk of exposure to Covid."

- Chapter 52 -

Max and Elizabeth watched the pandemic with interest. The lockdown provided the perfect excuse for them to cocoon together. They had been exposed to many infectious diseases over the course of their careers and were content to sit this one out. They walked Buckeye twice daily, ordered food from the grocery store and nearby restaurants, and enjoyed shopping on the Internet. The lockdown presented a novelty to them after their busy careers. In the evenings they would relax in the blue stuffed chairs in their bedroom, share a glass of wine, argue about current affairs, reminisce about former patients, discuss past mistakes, and envision their future together. They never ran out of things to banter about; often exclaiming, "My, how we suffer" as they relished the oasis they created.

Elizabeth and Max considered themselves honeymooners, but this honeymoon differed from the honeymoons they both experienced with their respective spouses so many years previously. Sex had lost its allure. It now required effort and planning with their old, aching and creaky bodies. Youthful passion and desire had been replaced though, with total acceptance and love. Not a bad tradeoff.

Elizabeth complained that the dialysis machine in her living room ruined her décor, but she enjoyed the visual harmony of Max sitting in the reading chair. Max assisted with Elizabeth's dialysis treatments as they played chess, read books, or watched movies. They discovered that the advertised two-hour dialysis sessions were, in fact, four-hour sessions with the preparation, set up and tear down of the machine. But they were retired, and time had lost its dominion.

Becky and Joe's wedding needed to be postponed several times as the lockdown dragged on and wedding venues closed. They gave up and got married over Zoom with friends and family, and a justice of the peace officiating. Not exactly as they had planned, but things were what they were. Their wedding would make a great story for their children and grandchildren.

Elizabeth often called Rachel to make sure she was surviving in the trenches. Rachel moaned and complained as she told the stories of her days. Elizabeth reminded Rachel that the pandemic was temporary and that all things are passing. She reassured her that she was strong and smart, and that she loved her.

Every day, Max and Elizabeth logged on to medical research sites to keep up with the latest research about the spread of Covid and its potential treatments. They'd watch TV and laugh at how the media misinterpreted and sensationalized the new developments.

One day, as Max scoured the internet during Elizabeth's dialysis session, he groaned and put his head in his hands.

Elizabeth looked up from her book. "What is it? What happened?"

"I stumbled upon some conspiracy websites. They mock and contradict research findings so far. For starters, they claim that no one is really dying, that doctors are falsely claiming Covid as a cause of death, on death certificates so hospitals can make more money. They want to convince people that Covid is fake, and the government is just trying to control people."

Elizabeth moaned. "What an insult to the integrity of doctors. What's going to happen if these websites spread and attain the status of truth?"

"I'm afraid they already have. Read some of this shit, Eli. They've created an entire universe of alternative facts."

"Alternative facts?"

"Lies." Max brought his laptop over for Eli to look at. "Opinions are malleable, and knowledge changes, but facts are facts. They're making up new facts, contradicting the ones they don't like."

"Oh, dear." She shook her head as she looked at the different websites. "They look so professional, a serious work of deception." Elizabeth clucked her tongue. "Definitely adds another level of confusion and darkness to the pandemic. Mark Twain once said, 'A lie travels halfway around the world before the truth has its boots on.'"

"My dear, I think it was Winston Churchill who said it."

"Well, whoever said it, knew the problems that lies cause. I don't know why anyone would prefer lies to the truth."

Max replied. "That's easy. Lies and conspiracy theories are a simple answer to a complex reality. The simpler the lie, the easier to sway people."

Elizabeth became obsessed with the disinformation, misinformation, and conspiracy theories saturating the internet, convinced that they were more dangerous than Covid. *Lies destroy trust; can destroy a society. Look at what happened in Rwanda.*

Max was more irritated with the CDC and public health websites for not explaining to the non-medical person how science in public health works, preparing readers for ambiguities and shifting recommendations as new data emerges. He believed that the unknowns and fears about Covid incited the development of conspiracy theories.

Elizabeth felt the problem was not public health communications per se, but the internet. "It spreads lies and disinformation. We know what we know because we have worked in health care our whole lives, but someone who hasn't, cant tell the difference between a lie and true public health information. They learn to distrust truth because of the thousands of lies disputing it."

- Chapter 53 -

The governor kept extending the lockdown as cases and deaths surged despite the draconian measures. The predicted few weeks turned into months, month after long, lonely month. Rachel and Darnell's FaceTime conversations encompassed everything, including the books they were reading and thoughts they were thinking. Rachel updated Darnell on the happenings in the dialysis unit, keeping the names confidential of course. He hated to admit that he craved dialysis unit gossip. Often, they argued about Covid and the lockdown restrictions.

Even with the arguments and the forces separating them, Darnell and Rachel found creative ways to care for each other. Darnell cooked meals (without pork) for Rachel and left them at her door with tender letters and scribbled pictures from his nephews on the lids of the casserole dishes. Rachel returned the empty dishes with love notes of her own and ordered toys and games from Amazon to help Darnell entertain the twins. The twins would leap and squeal when they discovered another brown cardboard box at the door of Darnell's apartment.

The twins' daycare center reopened; Cleveland State ended for the summer, but the Cash Flash Pawn shop remained closed. Darnell found himself the recipient of great swaths of empty time. He spent his days exploring Northeast Ohio on Rusty. Often, he'd stop to sit on a park bench, hoping to feel God's presence like he felt when he was dying. He felt nothing except a restless hunger. He found faith difficult and strange.

He'd ask God why He hid himself and argued with him that it made much more sense for him to reveal himself openly with a few miracles scattered here and there. "More people would believe in You." He watched people driving their cars or walking by and considered the stories of their lives. *I guess even one person's life is a miracle.*

In August, Shanita contracted Covid. She was sicker than she had ever been in her life. She spent her days in bed, too sick to watch TV, febrile, and coughing, trying to breathe. Her sons stayed with Darnell, sleeping with him in his bed.

Until Shanita caught Covid, Darnell believed that Covid was overrated and over-hyped. But as he watched her coughing and struggling to breathe, fearful that she would die, he developed a new respect for the invisible virus. Darnell dreaded losing his sister. His heart ached. After losing Will in January, he couldn't fathom losing Shanita too. He checked on her at least three times a day with his mask on, yelling through the door of her apartment. He dropped off cough medicine, a pulse oximeter, a thermometer, elderberry syrup, Tylenol, popsicles, and soup. He dropped off anything and everything he could imagine. He always asked about the results of her pulse oximeter reading, prepared to drive her to the hospital if it went lower than ninety. The twins stood at his side in the doorway and yelled, "We wuv you Mama," and left scribbled get-well cards that Darnell had helped them design.

His stomach churned with anxiety and dread. Darnell entertained the twins during those anxious weeks exploring the beach along Lake Erie. They waded in the water, built sand-castles, and played with shovels and dump trucks. He hugged them especially close when they read books together, some-times with tears in his eyes. He wrestled and played with them as if there would be no tomorrow. It took weeks, but gradu-ally, inch by inch, Shanita recovered, and the twins returned to day-care.

- Chapter 54 -

Sometimes when Rachel was home, Darnell would stop by to pick up his motorcycle in her garage. He occasionally knocked on Rachel's door, hoping she'd change her mind about quarantining. Even though she hungered for his touch, she'd wave at him through the front window and blow him a kiss. As she watched him drive away, her heart sank in misery.

The pandemic days in the dialysis unit continued to be relentless. The traditional animosity and divisions between the techs and nurses disappeared. They needed each other to survive each day, working side by side and sharing the burdens. Rachel was still responsible for supervising the techs, administering all the meds, and completing the documentation, on top of all the other work she had taken on.

One busy day, Rachel overheard Tamika coughing. She sent her home and encouraged her to take good care of herself, hoping it was just a cold and not Covid. Tamika never returned. Rachel found out from her family that she had been hospitalized with Covid and subsequently died in ICU with her children saying goodbye to her over FaceTime.

That night, during their FaceTime conversation, Rachel wept when she told Darnell that Tamika died from Covid. Through her sobs, she said, "I keep turning my head, expecting to see her face, and hear her voice, but she's gone. The unit isn't the same without her."

"I'd expect you to miss Tamika like you'd miss a bad toothache. She was always bad-mouthing you."

"I know…In the beginning she was like that. We got used to each other, I guess. We could have become good friends if given the time." Rachel said through her tears. "When

I think of her children without their mother, I can't stop weeping."

September arrived and Rachel celebrated Rosh Hashanah at her kitchen table over Zoom. What a year it had been. Once again, she recited the Unetanah Tokef with the congregation, naming all the ways a person can die, including some by plague. She didn't need to be reminded of her mortality and vulnerability this year, knowing in her bones how fragile and uncertain life is.

She considered the continuing lockdown and decided that perhaps life and death really are in God's hands, the government's hands, not so much. *Maybe we don't have the control over life and death that we think we have.* The lockdowns had made sense in the beginning, but they dragged on too long and people continued getting sick and dying of Covid. She wondered if the pandemic would have been worse without the lockdowns. Impossible to know. She knew for certain the lockdowns isolated people from each other and created fear. Fear and isolation kill people too. She knew people were working on a vaccine, but she expected that to take years.

She missed Darnell. During her long, lonely days, she read poetry. One line from a poem by Rumi, entitled Gambling, kept echoing in her heart: 'Gamble everything for love, if you're a true human being.' She didn't know how much time she had left to live, but wanted her days to be filled with love. She was tired of the lockdown, tired of Covid, and tired of trying so hard to do the right thing, whatever that was.

When Shanita had Covid, she had agonized about Darnell catching it, but when he didn't catch a sniffle even with his nephews sleeping in his bed, she rationalized that she didn't present such a danger to him, especially since she was so careful with precautions. She and Darnell could quarantine from the rest of the world together.

Rachel called Darnell and invited him over. When he arrived fifteen minutes later, she held him tightly and listened to his beating heart. "I can't live apart from you anymore. My heart is breaking. Let's go watch the leaves fall."

He smiled as he ran his fingers through her hair.

"They're not falling, my love; they've just started changing colors. Let's do a few other things while we wait."

Rachel snuggled into him, tenderly patted the tattoo on his arm, and whispered, "This moment only once. We could both be gone tomorrow. Now is our chance at life."

Appendix

<u>Dialysis accesses</u>

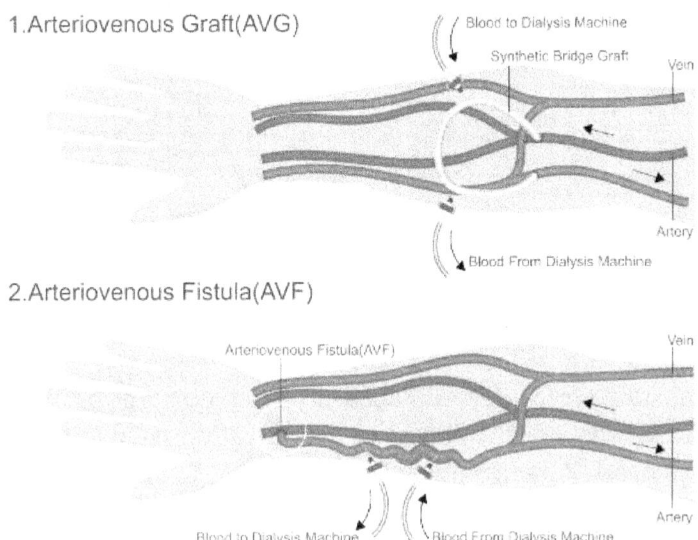

1. Arteriovenous Grafts (AVG)

If a person's arteries and veins aren't strong enough to support a fistula, tubes called grafts can be placed connecting an artery to a vein. Needles are placed into grafts as if it were the patient's own vein.

2. Arteriovenous Fistula (AVF)

Surgeons create fistulas by attaching an artery to a vein. Because the vein now has a larger flow of blood through it, it develops into a big vessel that's easy to insert needles in and provides the blood flow necessary for dialysis. This is the preferred access because it lasts the longest with the least risk of infection.

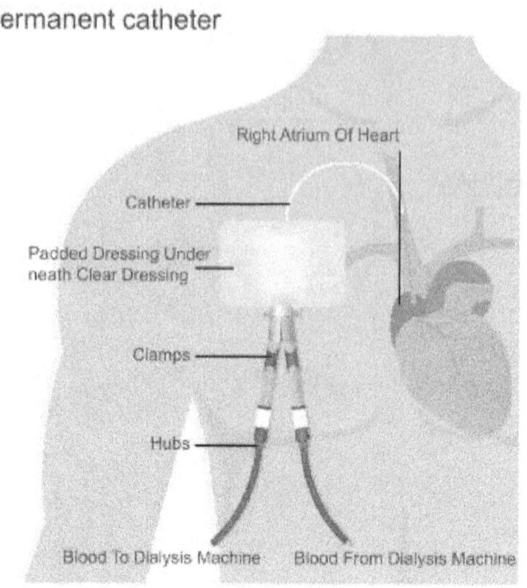

3. Permanent catheter or permcaths

Permcaths are catheters placed in the large vein that drains into a person's heart. The tip of a permcath rests in the atrium of the heart. Patients love permcaths because they don't have to get stuck with needles for dialysis. However, healthcare professionals hate them because they are dangerous. They can cause life-threatening infections in people's hearts, spines, joints, and brains.

Endnotes

[1] Alexander, Shauna (1962). Dialysis: they decide who lives, who dies. Life Magazine. November 9, 102–115.

[2] Blagg, C.R. (2007) The Early History of Dialysis for Chronic Renal Failure in the United States: A View from Seattle. American Journal of Kidney Diseases. 49 (3), 482–496.

<u>Dialysis information resources</u>

https://pmc.ncbi.nlm.nih.gov/articles/PMC4124935/

https://www.kidney.org/kidney-topics/hemodialysis

https://www.niddk.nih.gov/health-information/kidney-disease/
kidney-failure/hemodialysis

Topics and Questions
for Discussion

1. What do you think of Elizabeth's decision to forgo dialysis? Do you agree with Elizabeth that sometimes in health care we do things just because we can? What would you choose?

2. Do you think Harriet's choice to stop dialysis and throw herself a going away party was a form of assisted suicide? Can you imagine throwing a going away party for yourself?

3. After Max told Elizabeth's daughters about her plans to forgo dialysis, he told Elizabeth that sometimes a person has to break a law to do the right thing. Do you agree? Are there times in your life when you have made similar choices or wish you did?

4. Nurses are harder on each other for infractions and mistakes than physicians are on their peers. Why do you think that is? What is your explanation of Ms Legit's harshness toward Rachel?

5. There are two near death experiences described in this novel. Have you had one personally or heard of similar stories?

6. The author has witnessed numerous love affairs occur among dialysis patients and between patients and staff. How and why do you think this happens?

7. The author describes characters' experiences during Covid. What were yours like?

8. What kind of difficulties do you imagine Rachel and Darnell might encounter if they marry and start a family?

Acknowledgments

It takes a village to create a novel. Thank you to all the readers who commented on the early drafts: Jac Pearl, Toddra Liddell, Beverly Kimball, Lisa Sharon, Dick McCormick, Don Reed, Brett Barkley, Nancy Buchler, Janel Williams, Janet Fuchs, David Busch, Allison Hall, Kimberly Horka, Art Busch, Lora Bear, Mark Semer, Anne Meier Pryzbylkowski, Gail McGory, Susan Terkel, Robin Selinger.

About the Author

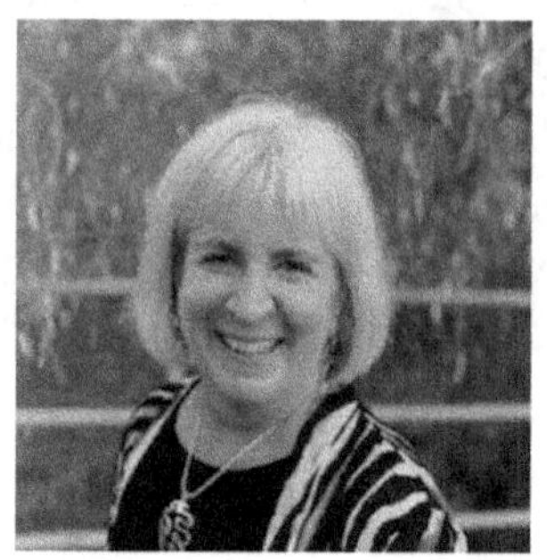

Susan Ellison Busch is a nurse practitioner, educator, and author. Her clinical specialty is nephrology. She has spoken at national conferences on topics related to dialysis and 22q.11 Deletion syndrome. Her first book, *Yearning for Normal*, a memoir about raising a son with 22q.11 Deletion Syndrome, is a Reader's Favorite Book Award Winner. She is the mother of three sons. Susan lives with her husband on the edge of the Cuyahoga Valley National Park in Ohio. When she isn't writing, she enjoys the trees and the sky, hiking, and playing tennis.